STUPID

The Hormone Weight Loss Solution

—

Fix your CRAZY Hormones and Finally Lose Weight for Good!

Jennifer Jolan & Rich Bryda

ISBN: 1477540113

ISBN13: 978-1477540114

CONTENTS

ABOUT THE AUTHORS

Jennifer Jolan is a best-selling author and "America's Weight Loss Queen."

Over 120,000 people have read her How to Lose Weight Spinning Around in a Circle Like Kids book. Thousands more have bought her best-selling 1-Day Diet: The Fastest "Diet" in the World book which can be found on Amazon.com.

In addition, she has written over 1,100 articles about weight loss, and has helped thousands of people around the world fix their weight problems without starvation, restrictive dieting, or struggle.

Rich Bryda is the best-selling author of The Effortless Exercise System for Men and a sought after nutrition consultant and fitness coach who is known for his cutting-edge exercise and dieting advice and breaking it down into simple, easy-to-digest, and practical tips for everyone from beginners to advanced athletes.

INTRODUCTION

We've all ridden the diet merry-go-round. Some of us have done so far too many times.

Round and round we go, and when we stop we're back to the weight we began... or higher.

If you're tried diet after diet you're not alone. Although we've now taught tens of thousands of our readers and clients how to lose weight and keep it off, we didn't have the answers at the start. Or in the middle either! It took combined years of research, study, trial, error, and working with and researching the best minds in the business to optimize our bodies' weight and create a lifestyle that enables us to keep it off without effort.

But it is possible to be healthy, be fit, and feel great. That is, *if* you understand that your hormones are the regulators that work for you or against you. Hormones stop your weight loss or add to your weight loss. They keep you healthy or allow you to deteriorate. As your hormones go so goes your health.

If you want to understand a better approach than a diet merry-go-round, you've come to the right place.

Jennifer Jolan & Rich Bryda

CHAPTER 1

HEALTH IS THE KEY, NOT WEIGHT

The key to losing weight and *keeping* it off is not found in any diet on earth. The key to losing weight and *keeping* it off isn't any eating plan in existence today.

The key to losing weight and keeping it off is two-fold:

1. Fix your health

2. Live a healthy lifestyle

Your body is a regulating machine. Your body knows its optimum weight. In spite of bad weight experiences you've maybe had in the past, your body *does* always want to get to its optimum weight as quickly as it can. A well-oiled machine works tirelessly and when your body is the equivalent of a well-oiled machine it will work for you in ways you never dreamed. But until you oil it – that is, until you fix your health and adopt a lifelong healthy eating and health regimen – your body is not going to be able to work with you. Your body will work against you.

The result of our bodies working against us is the overweight condition we often find ourselves in. This multiplies into severe health problems later. We focus too much on the symptom and not the real problem. The problem is not the fat stored on our thighs, hips, and around our waists. Our bodies simply don't have the ability to stay at an optimum weight when we don't correct our control center.

Do you know what your body uses to control weight loss or weight gain? Your body uses the same mechanisms to control your weight that it uses to control how you feel at any given moment, how you look, how your skin feels, how active you are, how much sex you desire, how much you sleep, how effectively you think and communicate, and scores of other factors. Primarily, your body uses hormones as triggers to turn on and off every aspect of your well-being.

We're going to help you balance your hormones and health. Maximizing your hormones *before* focusing on weight loss will produce results you might find amazing. Once you fix your hormones, weight loss will be an easy and a natural result. Treat the problem (your messed up hormones) and not the symptoms (your extra weight).

> **Note:** Sometimes, malnutrition and bad brain nutrients and imbalanced hormones can put you into a state of starvation even though you are eating a lot. If you are underweight and want to bump up your pounds, don't focus on eating more. Focus on getting your brain and hormones, your body's central control panel switches, where they should be. Your body will then be freed up to get your weight to a more optimal level.

By the way, as you begin to stabilize your hormone balances to healthy levels, your weight will not be the first thing to be fixed by your newly healthy body. Your digestion, sleep patterns, energy levels, and strength will probably improve first. Once your body has adjusted properly to its new turbo-charged hormone levels the weight will begin to drop consistently soon after.

Hormones Control Your Health, Your Brain Controls Your Hormones and Other Things

To put yourself into the best shape you've ever been, you *must* focus on your body's regulators. Those are your key hormones that need to be in balance.

There is another factor to consider too. Besides your hormones, you must also get your brain into balance. Even if you consider yourself a clear thinker, that doesn't mean that your brain's nutrients are in their optimal state and balance.

We've written about putting your brain's nutrients into balance in *Brain Controlled Weight Loss - The Solution to Failed Diets & Exercise Programs!*, a book that you owe it to yourself to read along with this one. We're not mentioning our brain book as a cheap plug; if we didn't stand behind it so strongly we wouldn't have written this or told you about it. We're telling you this so you'll understand that it is your brain that actively controls your various body's reactions and hormone triggers.

When you have an imbalance in your brain's primary chemicals and neurotransmitters, you must correct that imbalance immediately. Otherwise your brain won't be fully freed up to handle what it was designed to do. If you're overweight and tired, an out-of-balance brain needs to be looked into and fixed first before focusing on pure weight loss. If you don't, your weight loss will be temporary at best and can possibly work *against* your overall health.

It's critical that you focus both on your brain's chemical nutrients and your body's hormone balances. For decades, books, trainers, and nutritionists have focused on the symptom – being overweight – and not the regulators and controllers of the symptom – hormones and the brain's chemical nutrients. Recent revelations about the brain and hormone balances have produced astounding results when it comes to people's health and weight levels.

It's so very true that we cannot emphasize it enough: Fix your hormones and brain nutrients and you'll fix your health… AND lose weight!

When Things Are Severe

Obviously, some people have severe health problems that must be addressed immediately, such as Multiple Sclerosis and Alzheimer's issues. We are not saying that bringing the hormones and brain back into balance will fix those overnight or ever.

But so many times, the symptoms of those severe diseases and other maladies such as hypertension and high cholesterol can be caused by hormone imbalances. At the very least hormone, brain nutrient, vitamin, and mineral deficiencies can contribute to the start of such maladies and perhaps even are instrumental in keeping those problems active.

No matter where you are on the healthy/unhealthy meter if you repair your hormones you will at the *least* begin to stop contributing to other problems hampered by hormone imbalances. And at best you may see reversals. Your hormones will be able once again to regulate your body and your brain will once again be able to regulate your hormones and other activities.

Hormonal Balance is Pure Health

If you fail to believe that serious issues *can* be addressed through a non-medicinal look at your body, your hormones, your brain, and your lifestyle, you owe it to yourself to watch the following astounding video by Dr. Terry Wahls. A few years ago, her Multiple Sclerosis reached the tipping point so much so that her MS confined her to a wheelchair for four years until she began systematically reversing her MS and actually repaired her brain's myelin sheathing (the insulation around the brain's pathways).

Her video is here (and if you know anything about MS this will amaze you): http://kaleuniversity.org/5103-multiple-sclerosis-dr-wahls

Dr. Wahls now spends her days bike-riding and skiing and has been symptom-free from MS just 18 months after focusing on a non-medicinal lifestyle which fixed her brain, hormones, and MS through diet alone. Remember, she was an invalid just a couple of years earlier, confined to a wheelchair without a decent quality of life.

The FDA, USDA, AMA, AOA, and all the others in the governmental and medical alphabet soups, all with vested interests to sell you drugs and keep your food intake unhealthy to maintain their constant customer flow, made it illegal to be told by a non-licensed practitioner that you can often fix your health problems through non-medicinal purposes. That is why we leave it up to Dr. Wahls to convince you in her video.

We are not rallying against drug corporations and the free market. We're not rallying against government either. We *are* rallying against the government/corporate connections in place. If only food and drugs *were* available in a free-market and not regulated by the FDA.

With the FDA and other advisory groups like them, as movies such as *Fat Head* (wonderful movie and funny too!), *King Corn*, and *Food, Inc.* have shown so clearly, the foxes are guarding the hen house. The very company executives who have vested interests in growing corn and other grains that your body was never designed to ingest, and the drug company officials who want you to buy their drugs, are *advisors for the FDA*. I'd be happy if there was a wall of separation but there is none.

> **Note:** Have you ever asked yourself why the *Food* and the *Drug* regulators are the same group? Shouldn't they be at odds with one another? Should food officials want you to eat *such healthy food that you'll never get sick or need drugs?* That's not what we have. It almost leads one to conclude that the food and drug parts of the FDA work together to ensure that one provides customers for the other.

Always remember: if you focus on food and weight without the vision of fixing your body's control systems, you may lose weight temporarily but your body is going to halt your weight loss eventually and revert back to storing weight. Your body simply won't have the ability or freedom to regulate your weight properly.

Stop Your Moaning By Fixing Your Hormones

It turns out that if you want real results to appear on your hips and thighs you must take care of your body's regulators. Those are your hormones! Ultimately, the health of your body depends on the health of your hormones.

Sure, it's possible to starve yourself by reducing your ingested calories down to an extremely low level and you'll lose weight. Maybe. For a while at least. You lose weight because you literally starve your body and it must begin to cannibalize itself including your muscles and whatever lean tissue mass you happen to have. But on most calorie-restrictive lifestyles you and your health will go away as quickly as the fat. Only the fat will return.

You must here and now make a promise to yourself: Assuming we convince you that the proper brain fuel produces the best body results possible, and we will, your goal from this point forward should be to focus not on your thighs but on your hormones *first*. (Again, you need to understand the vital role that your brain's chemicals play too. For that, see *Brain Controlled Weight Loss - The Solution to Failed Diets & Exercise Programs!*.)

You've been sold a bill of goods all your life when you've been told that to lose weight and build lean muscle mass, get more energy, and feel better, that you have to fix your caloric intake.

Not so.

To the extent you've happened to balance some hormones in the past through eating, you may have accomplished some of those goals. Nevertheless, since you didn't realize the prime importance of focusing on your hormone regulators first then you didn't accomplish your goals as fully as you could have. And if you're like most of us, you didn't stay lean or feel good for long. Because you weren't taught that your hormones are the regulators of how much you weigh and how good you feel.

Weight control isn't about calories – weight control is all about hormones.

CHAPTER 2

WHAT EXACTLY IS A HORMONE?

If you've read anything about hormones in the past you may have been left with more questions than answers.

One of the reasons so many people get confused when told about hormones, especially given how much press hormones have been getting lately, is that the fundamentals aren't explained. Until you understand the basics, you have less reason to accept or believe that hormone balance will play such a large role in your health and weight loss.

It's the goal of this book to make hormones as easy to understand as possible. You don't need to know micro-biology to understand the fundamentals or hormones. You don't need a degree in Health Sciences to realize how vital that hormones are to every aspect of your body. We aren't going to go in-depth into charts and graphs and diagrams of the functions of hormones.

Who cares about all that if you're not in school? You just want to know how to get healthy and achieve your optimum weight, right?

All that takes is understand just the basics of hormones and then you need to learn ways to put your key hormones into balance.

The Importance of Hormone Regulation in Weight Loss

Most will read this book because they want to lose weight. That is a fine reason. We're told that obesity is at epidemic proportions. This is true.

Decades of the American government putting fat and protein at the top of the USDA's Food Pyramid has resulted in scores of fat-free products on every aisle at every grocery store in the nation and the world. By eliminating fat in food, we've become a grossly-fat nation. By eliminating protein and replacing it with dangerous levels of grains and body-damaging faux food such as soy, we have become a nation of people who are obese and unhealthy.

> **Note:** Just in case that wasn't clear, let's make it abundantly clear: eliminating fat from your food *increases* fat on your thighs, hips, and belly. Not one objective study has shown otherwise. Did you know farmers give calves skim milk to fatten them up? Even worse, low-fat milk is a likely source of infertility among women according to a recent Harvard study. Whole (and raw) milk is the way nature intends milk to be… with lots of fat. If you are overweight, your hormones are almost certainly out of whack. One of the ways to correct that is to *add fat to your diet*. The type of fat you add matters but in general it is the fat you've been told for 40 years not to consume – animal fat – that is some of the best fat sources available to help you lose weight. To clarify further so we're on the same page, the grains and

abundance of fruit and starchy vegetables you've been told to make the largest part of your family's diet is making America fat and unhealthy. The bottom line is this: The Food Pyramid (shown below) is a lie.

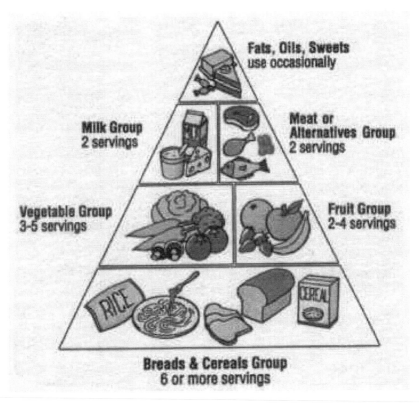

It's not just America suffering from an obesity epidemic although we started seeing the results of the FDA's advice first. We've exported the dangerous notion of a grain-rich, no-fat diet to other nations. Nations who never had high incidences of obesity- and dietary-related health problems such as diabetes and hypertension are seeing those numbers spike like never before.

The beat goes on. Just this week the government announced additional plans to replace good protein and fat sources in school lunch programs with grains and dried fruits and (the worst) fruit juices. School children can expect more health problems as a result. Their hormones will be even more out of balance as they consume more and more obesity-creating "food."

Fruit is a Great Example of a Bad Solution

It can't be stated enough: You need to focus on making your body's regulators – your hormones – happy and ignore the government regulators who want you fat. If that sounds like a harsh accusation, there is no other conclusion which can be drawn given the abundance of data that shows a low-fat, high grain diet is deadly.

The abuse of fruit by government-approved dieticians is a perfect example. Fruit in moderation is great. Fruit contains antioxidants and eating a variety of fruit of various colors throughout the week, with an extra emphasis on low-glycemic berries over higher-impact sugary fruits such as oranges and bananas, gives you nutrition your body needs.

But fruit today is often promoted in quantities that can't help but end up replacing good animal and nut proteins and fats. Eating fruit the way it comes off the tree or vine (and organically grown *every* time you can get it) is a fantastic way to get some nutrients that your body – and hormones – love! Eating dried fruit (sold in schools now instead of candy bars) (producing the same miserable results but don't taste as good) removes the water which makes you feel full and leaves you wanting more. Fruit juice is hardly better than full-calorie soda pop; tons of fructose sugar without any of the fiber to slow down the sugar's toxic effects.

> **Note:** Both diet *and* regular sodas contain a preservative called *benzoate* to help maintain freshness. Benzoate interacts with your body's Vitamin C and breaks down to benzene which is suspected to be a carcinogen.

Dr. Joseph Mercola, MD, had this to say about fruit consumption in a recent newsletter to his readers:

> In the past many have objected to my position on limiting fruit intake and I am fine with that, BUT if you are convinced, for whatever reason, that you can have unlimited fruits than I would strongly encourage you to have a blood uric acid level drawn. High uric acid is a potent marker for fructose toxicity, so if your levels are above:
>
> - 4 mg/dl for men
>
> - 3.5 mg/dl for women
>
> ... then you would be wise to avoid all forms of fructose until your levels have normalized—just as you would with high insulin levels.

4mg or 3.5 mg of fructose is a surprisingly low amount. You don't even have to get your fructose toxicity measured if you've bought into the lie that you need multiple servings of fruit and fruit juice daily. If you've followed the FDA's advice on that, get off the toxic bandwagon now and just say *no* to fruit for a while until your system gets better balanced. Eat plenty of fibrous and colorful vegetables for your vitamins and minerals that you don't get from the rest of your diet.

> **Note:** Some tell us they worry about vitamin C deficiency when we discuss fruit with them. If you want to ensure adequate amounts of C from food alone, tomatoes and other veggies have it but also you don't have to give up the C and other vitamins from citrus fruit as long as you stick to limes and lemons for a while. One lime has statistically zero grams of fructose and a lemon has less than 1 gram. They both offer the advantage that they reduce the glycemic load of other food you eat so if you squeeze a lime or lemon over your chicken and broccoli tonight, you'll reduce that small amount of carbs down even further plus you'll get the C you worry about.

> **Note:** Other extremely low fructose fruits include cranberries, passion fruit, and prunes. Slightly higher but probably still safe even for a current fruit addict trying to kick the habit, passion fruit, guava, dates, raspberries, blackberries, star fruit, kiwifruit, a clementine, up to ten cherries, and a cup of strawberries all weigh in at low levels of fructose and would be okay bridges to help ease you out of your sugar addiction without reducing your daily fruit consumption entirely.

One of the ways you put your hormones into balance is through your diet. It turns out as no surprise that the food and supplements that help balance your hormones are the very food and supplements that help you lose weight too. Along the way, you not only are decreasing your intake of fat-causing food but you are increasing your intake of hormone-balancing food. Your weight loss will explode over whatever results you might get if you focus only on calories because your hormones will begin activating your weight loss in a full-steam-ahead manner.

We'll talk a lot more about fruit throughout this book, especially in Chapter 4 where we cover a hormone-healthy diet and lifestyle. Fruit isn't off limits at all. But you must approach fruit wisely as you do with all your food to ensure healthy hormones.

Your machine – your body – will be well-oiled and functioning lean and mean.

How Much Fiber is Enough?

Fiber is vital to keep food flowing through your body the way it should. It's been said that one needs from 40 to 50 grams of fiber daily to stay regular. This is a general rule of thumb but there is one even better.

If you are honest with yourself that you truly have regular, healthy, good stools on a regular basis, you almost certainly get enough fiber. Your gut will react to too much or too little and you'll be the first to know if something is up. Don't let an occasional problem day or two guide you. Long-term regularity is a sure sign that you don't need to fix anything in that area.

Long-term bowel movement problems indicate a sure sign that you need to address your gut.

Probiotics, fermented food, and more fiber is almost always the trio in short supply when gut problems are present. Still, too much fiber can cause loose stools also. If you've been supplementing with fiber and haven't seen many good results, stop the supplementation and try to maintain a good level of fibrous veggies, seeds, and nuts for a week or two to see if anything changes. If not, you certainly should see a physician to make sure there is nothing else going on that should be addressed medically.

Hormones 101

Let's keep this section short, shall we?

You want answers not science. Although the underlying science is actually fun for us, we don't want to waste your time. We want to give you answers that will balance key hormones and put your weight optimization into full gear.

The system in your body that contains your hormones is collectively called your *endocrine system.*

A hormone is a chemical in your body. Usually, a hormone is created or generated in one part of your body by an organ and sent to another part of your body to do a job. Many hormones perform multiple jobs. Many of your body's hormones, or chemicals, can regulate multiple activities. Our glandular system is primarily responsible for hormone creation although we can generate some of our needed hormones elsewhere such in our stomach. Our cells can produce hormones too which then regulate other cells.

Examples of organs that can create hormones in bodies are:

- Ovaries

- Testes

- Thyroid Gland

- Pituitary Gland

The bottom line is this: a hormone is a specific chemical that helps regulate a part or parts of your body. The regulation might be physical such as sexual functioning or it might seem to be more of a chemical regulation such as metabolism.

Hormones often allow for free-flowing or blocked communication and bodily responses. If you are low on a hormone, the organ or cells or chemical that hormone is supposed to regulate or communicate with will be out of balance and not work optimally.

Your body contains, produces, and acts upon many different hormones. Several hundred hormones run around in your system as a matter of fact.

There is not one key hormone although some hormones play more important and active roles than others. In this book we will focus on the hormones that help the typical body get and stay healthy and get and stay lean.

> **Note:** Some hormones, such as insulin, control other hormones.

Sources of Hormones

As said, your body usually creates hormones. A healthy, vibrant body creates a good balance of needed hormones.

Through various actions and sources such as supplementation and prescriptions you can add certain hormones to your body through non-natural means. This is not in and of itself bad although many sources and methods for increasing certain hormones have been flawed through the years. Some synthetic hormones are used in *hormone replacement therapy* effectively while others have been found to be dangerous and produce unexpected results.

A healthy body with all the right ingredients in place will generally produce a healthy array of hormones that work in tandem and are in balance. As we age, our hormone generation can decrease. This can be okay depending on the hormone and your response and needs. For others, adding back hormones as aging occurs can be a big benefit through synthetic hormone replacement or a newer method called bio-identical hormone replacement, which replace specific hormones with identical chemical structure to the same hormones created by your body as opposed to a synthetic hormone which differs at the chemical level from a 100% naturally-produced hormone.

Diseases find it far more difficult to manifest themselves in your body when your hormones are in balance. It can't be said enough times: focusing on hormonal balance, perhaps for the first time in your life, means you will be healthier and your weight will be far easier to control than if you let your hormones get out of balance.

A Quick Introductory Example

Not every hormone we're going to discuss here relates to weight loss directly but they all relate indirectly in some way.

For example, there is a hormone that regulates how well you sleep. If you aren't sleeping well, you'll learn ways to help improve that hormone's imbalance. The hormone is melatonin.

Melatonin is important because sleep is important for health reasons. Without adequate sleep we are at risk emotionally with those we live and work with because we are more apt to be cranky when we are tired. A lack of sleep makes us less effective at work so our work suffers and ultimately our productivity can suffer from long-term insomnia enough to affect future advancement. Long-term fatigue makes us susceptible to illness through a deterioration of our immune systems.

The hormone melatonin is critical for weight loss even though melatonin's primary job is to regulate sleep. As the October 5, 2010 *Annals of Internal Medicine* explains, dieters who got adequate sleep lose twice the amount of body fat that they lost when their sleep was restricted. In addition, with inadequate amounts of sleep the dieters felt far hungrier due to an imbalance in the ghrelin hormone, a hormone that regulates hunger.

Given this initial example, when we cover hormones throughout this book that don't directly seem to impact your weight loss, please know that they do impact your weight loss *indirectly* at the least. And don't you want to stack the odds in your favor every step of the way with losing weight? Don't you want to maximize and optimize your body's weight loss? Certainly you do and so all of the hormones discussed here play an important role in your health and weight. In addition, if a hormone relates to your body's overall health, such as your thyroid, there is no way your body is going to be able to focus on optimizing your weight if it's dealing with an imbalance in its thyroid.

Your body is an amazing, multi-processing machine that works on many activities at once. But your body can get stressed out when forced to deal with problem areas that you could otherwise eliminate. Balancing hormones is a fantastic and required way to ensure that any excess weight is dealt with effectively and as quickly as possible.

Dysfunctional Hormones

Hormones act dysfunctional when they are out of balance or not at their peak levels. Not only do organs and cells not communicate with each other effectively when your hormones are not at their peak levels, but some low hormone levels cause poor nutrient uptake in your body so you don't get the nutrition your body needs to function properly.

Hormone overloads can cause as much damage or more than low levels of hormones. For example, both estrogen and testosterone are present in healthy men and women. Obviously, the levels considered normal for one sex differs for the other sex.

Today we are experiencing far greater levels of estrogen due to pesticides in the soil and soy in food products. (Soy sauce is not a risk factor because the soy is fermented and doesn't cause the negative effects in men.) By the time you add up the amount of pesticides ingested from the non-organic foods we buy, we eat one pound of pesticides each year. From the start, the average American is being attacked with hormone-damaging food. We're going to be discussing food quite a bit in this book as well as food sources and the types of food that help align your hormonal balance instead of put your hormones out of sync.

The Bottom Line

Hormones control your sex drive. Hormones control how well you sleep. Hormones control your metabolism by determining whether food you eat should be used for energy right then or stored as fat. Hormones control when you are hungry and when you are full. If hormones regulate virtually every activity in your body including the ability or inability to lose weight, doesn't it make sense to get your hormones working at the best in order to get to your best weight possible?

Many diets address just one or two hormones whether or not they realize it. You need to concentrate on a series of primary hormones to help your health and then to lose weight and keep it off. In Jennifer's wildly popular weight loss volume entitled *1-Day Diet: The Fastest "Diet" in the World*, she doesn't even mention hormones. Yet, the diet is geared toward maximizing several key hormones and, using a few tricks, produces extremely quick results especially for those who have tried to lose weight in the past using more traditional diets such as calorie restrictive weight loss gimmicks.

Fixing your hormones not only will let you get and stay healthier but you should lose weight far more effectively as well.

CHAPTER 3

FOOD AND HORMONES

Sadly, many of our hormone problems come from man-made activities. It's not just a poor diet that can put our hormones out of balance. It's how we typically live as well.

The fault is not ours necessarily. Our society has become prosperous. Technology has developed new ways to do more with fewer resources. While some complain about how the "big box stores" produce shoddy merchandise, others realize that companies such as Wal-Mart sell lots of items to families who would never before be able to afford much of what they now get weekly. Is being able to buy your child a toy, even if it's not the quality an expensive one might be, better than giving her nothing on her birthday? Offering a wide range of economic choices enables far more people to participate in the economy and have a higher standard of living.

This prosperity comes with a price however. In getting more for less, in producing more using fewer resources, things slip along the way. Sadly, our health is often one of the casualties. The choices for lower-quality foods should still be available because some food is better than no food if you're starving. But the problem comes in when the government and its highest advisors from the food and drug companies all have financial incentives to keep you ignorant of good and bad choices.

The Food Supply

The term "organic" was unknown to our great-grandparents. They often grew most of what they ate. Their cattle and chickens and pigs were fed in part scraps from the table that would we might consider refuse. The table scraps that they couldn't feed to the pigs they would put in a box outside to produce compost to enrich the soil in the next set of crops. They used their chicken coop's waste product to fertilize and enrich soil used for new plantings. They would rotate crops to maintain a healthy blend of nutrients in the soil. Often their produce was so high in nutrients that pesticides were hardly a problem.

> **Note:** When plants have a high nutritional value, often called a *high-brix reading*, bugs that would otherwise eat the plants get diarrhea and die because their systems don't handle highly nutritious produce well.

A fully-functioning farm, sometimes today called a *permaculture* farm, utilized all resources in a closed system. Run-off water from one field was used to water another that was planted below it. The upper tier would need fresher water and the lower-tier getting the runoff had crops that grew better with the secondary water.

Organic and permaculture farming are buzzwords today that are treated as though they are some newfangled way of growing food. Your great grandparents didn't use the terms permaculture or organic or high-brix. They called it "farming" and "ranching" and "gardening."

Your great grandparents didn't worry about their food not being nutritious enough. It was nutritious enough. Sometimes, depending on the crop, theirs were many times more nutritious than what we can get at any traditional grocery store today.

We have paid the price in all the high pesticide, low-nutrient foods that we've eaten since our Moms were convinced to forgo breast feeding and give us "baby formula" and water in plastic bottles laced (only the label says "enhanced") with fluoride. We've paid the price in health problems that have become epidemic. Our hormones cannot keep up with the demands placed on them. Our bodies therefore cannot keep up.

Dr. Al Sears, MD, recently wrote this:

> [...] but today an apple a day is not going to do anything for you. The produce you get from your grocery store doesn't have the same level of vitamins, minerals or fiber it did years ago. In fact, you would have to eat 26 of today's apples to equal just one apple from 1914. (Source: Lindlahr, 1914: USDA 1963 and 1997.)
>
> Why should you care about that? Commercial farming has stripped our food of the very nutrients we need to stay vital, young and full of energy.
>
> Today's commercial farmers grow fruits and vegetables that are designed to look good on the shelf. That means they're often little more than pith and water. And harsh fertilizers leave the soil with few – if any – minerals to nourish the plants.
>
> Even the U.S. Department of Agriculture admits that vitamin and mineral levels have fallen by as much as 81

percent over the last 30 years. (Source: Vegetables without Vitamins," Life Extension Magazine March 2001.)

The Fake and Almost-Foods

It's all the fake foods we eat that causes people to get fat. People are living longer due to technical advances in items such as advanced heart devices but the quality of life is not increasing at the same rate. The extra years are not usually quality years.

The elderly are honestly asking themselves, "Why did they always call these the *golden years*?"

Eating organic produce and healthy meats and oils means that your body gets far more value with less food. Instead of eating non-food, or barely-food, you'll be eating real food that contains real nutrients and none of the cell-harming agents such as pesticides. Seek out local farmers and ranchers to get your food as close to home as possible. It is far fresher when it arrives.

> **Note:** If you find a good rancher who understands the importance of grass-fed beef with virtually no grains or lifelong antibiotics, see if you can purchase a half or whole beef when the rancher sends the cattle to slaughter. You will pay far less buying healthy meat in "bulk" like that than any other method and you'll get healthier meat. If you don't have any place to put it, go *now* to Best Buy and just buy a chest freezer. They are only a few hundred dollars and you'll have a place to put your beef and within a few buys, you'll have paid for the freezer in savings over what you would have paid the grocery store.

31

By the way don't overcook your meat no matter how good the charred outside tastes. (And it tastes pretty good to some of us!) The longer you cook most food, the more that food's nutritional value diminishes (except for tomatoes... they're actually healthier after slight cooking). As meat beings to char, carcinogens form and you'll therefore have more stuff that your body now has to deal with. For those of us who have gone from ordering extra-well done all our lives to medium rare now, we have found that those who used to tell us that meat had better taste the less it's cooked were telling us the truth. Plus, it's better for us too, so it's a double bonus.

Another caveat is to avoid cured meats, bacon, and sausage meats that contain nitrates and nitrites. You can find them at health food stores without the nitrates and nitrites. Even better, a local rancher might sell some to you without all that garbage that damages your hormones and cells.

Genetics and Hormones in Our Foods

Perhaps you've heard of *GMO* food. This is *genetically modified organism* (sometimes called *genetically engineered organism* or *GEO*). This is food that includes crops as well as animals that have been genetically modified. Supposedly since 1996 no animals are GMO in the food chain, although most animals are fed unnatural products that affect the way they grow and mature.

The goal of all this phony food modification is to grow a larger food supply in a smaller amount of time for less cost. That is a goal worthy of pursuing. By growing cheaper food at a faster rate we all can obtain food like never before in the history of the world. The problem is that these food modifications aren't limited to the developing countries that need all the help they can get to have a stable food supply so they can begin to prosper. The problem is that almost *all* food today contains some form of this modification.

The backlash has begun against companies using these tactics to change the way food is raised. Organic food was an attempt to limit or prevent the use of pesticides and genetic and hormone modification in food. Sadly, the label "organic" is loose enough to allow many things into our food that the originators of the term do not want. But on the whole, organic produce is far healthier for you and your family than non-organic.

> **Note:** Have you ever compared organic food to non-organic (called "conventional food") in the supermarkets that carry organic food? Often the organic food looks less healthy and goes old far faster once you get it home. Plus, it can be twice the cost. Who wants that? You should keep in mind a few things before forgoing the organic sections though because all is not always as it seems. First, food grown in a healthy environment is going to cost more. It also should *not* look better! Have you ever seen anything more beautiful than the perfect, beautiful apples as in the front bins of your grocery store? They are beautiful without blemish because the heavy pesticides kept every critter away for acres and the wax used to polish those apples makes them look better than a freshly-shined floor. Not having pesticides means that the organic produce might show a few signs of fatigue and perhaps initial bug attack here and there. Not having the cell-level modifications means they won't last as long as organic food because they haven't been laced with formaldehyde-like preservatives. They might only last as long as your great-grandparents' produce lasted. In other words, they are *normal, good-tasting, healthy*

ping to cost more if you want it. You can buy a
r made from pressed particle board or a more
r that will last far longer and be more
comfortable. Everything is a choice. Is your family worth
making the cheap choice when it comes to their health?

The Organic Label Can Be a Concern Too

By the way, your great grandparents would not even be able to
label their beef organic today. This is where some problems
arise with such labeling. Organic beef means that the cattle
never had antibiotics of any kind put in its system. But if your
great grandfather's cow got an infection, your great grandfather
would give the cow a shot of antibiotics and in 3 days the cow
would be great. Such specific use of antibiotics is fine and is a
long way from the antibiotic-laced food most cows are fed
today from cradle to grave to ward off dying as baby calves
since they are born, raised, and live in their own feces and fed
genetically-engineered corn their whole lives. Cattle were
designed to graze on grass in the fields and cows with that kind
of life produce healthy milk and beef.

So if you have a choice when it comes to your beef or chicken
or pork, grass-fed and cage-free is actually preferred over pure
organic. Smaller ranchers are beginning to understand this and
are offering grass-fed beef and free-range chicks and pork.
They avoid the term "organic" for their meats so they can get
the animal well with antibiotics, when needed… which is rare.
Otherwise, the animals roam the fields, eat the grass, the slop
and bugs (chickens love bugs and those that can free-range
during the daytime produce extremely healthy eggs and poultry
meat for your family).

If it all seems complicated, it is. It didn't used to be.

One way to decide what kind of food is healthiest is to think back to this chapter's premise: your great grandparents ate far healthier than we do today. If you run across a farmer or rancher who raises crops and meat the way your great grandparents would have done it, you've found a wonderful supply of food for your family. Forget the labels organic and permaculture and high-brix and just use common sense when considering your food source.

> **Note:** Google is your friend when you want to source quality food including healthy raw, whole milk. Even in the big cities, farms are often all around you that produce good food for the remnant such as those of us who want our apples to look normal but not necessarily perfect. We know that a perfect apple, as Eve found out soon enough, can be unusually deceptive!

Synergy – The Sum is Greater than the Individual Parts

Knowing all this helps your hormone levels in several ways. Your hormones need healthy and real food along with a few other commonsense things. They don't ask for much.

Sometimes exercise will boost a hormone. Sometimes a synthetic hormone is available when you cannot quite get enough help from food and exercise. (Sometimes synthetic hormones are bad too!) Sometimes a bio-identical hormone is available that is just like the hormones you produce at the cell level. Sometimes drugs will boost a needed hormone. Sometimes supplements will do so.

Our primary focus will be on the food you eat throughout the rest of this book. That is the very best way you can get your hormones into balance. That is also the very best way to feel

look your best. When supplements or a hormone
em has been found to be useful you'll read about
ough, food is going to be the prescription you
use here to balance your key hormones.

In the next chapter we're going to cover a simple, easy-to-follow hormone-healthy diet. Then in the rest of the book, we change gears and focus on one hormone at a time. All of these hormones affect your health in major ways and ultimately are crucial for keeping your weight off forever.

It's the nature of a book like this to focus on one topic at a time, such as one hormone per chapter as the next several chapters do. Still, while you are focusing on individual hormones, keep in mind that *we* will stay focused on your overall health. We will always offer food advice that not only will boost a specific hormone but also will boost others, or at least the food will not negatively affect the other hormones along the way. We will stay holistic even when discussing individual hormones.

If you are out of balance in one or more hormones, only a good doctor, one who understands the importance of hormones and natural eating and supplementation, will be able to tell you for certain. Look in the phone book or on Google for local doctors who offer *chelation therapy*. Those who do often are in tune with proper nutrition and can test for key hormones through a series of full-spectrum blood and saliva tests. These doctors are less likely than a traditional and typical doctor who tries to treat symptoms first with drugs or surgery before they treat the root causes such as hormone imbalances through diet.

Note: Always get a full spectrum blood test that tests for as many of the key hormones mentioned in the final chapters of this book as well as other health indicators such as sodium and potassium levels. If you accept a test that doesn't cover a full spectrum of hormones, you and your doctor are more likely to miss key connections between all your hormone levels that can help you zero-in on problems. Your physician must have knowledge of the way all your key hormones interact to properly evaluate any test results you get.

CHAPTER 4

A HEALTHY HORMONE DIET

Is there a general eating plan that will help balance your hormones *and* help you lose weight dramatically *and* get you feeling great?

The simple answer is yes.

This eating plan is not a diet. It is a lifelong style of eating that you and your family need to adopt.

Be warned: it takes guts because it goes against all that your government and most traditional doctors tell you. It goes against what many of your grocery store signs and processed food boxes tell you. It goes against what most restaurants call "healthy" on menus. It goes against most diets you've ever heard of.

How can all those authority sources be wrong? A better question is this: How can hundreds of millions of great-grandparents who lived well into their 90s all be wrong? The simple answer is they were not wrong. They were healthy and did not suffer from the plethora of maladies that affect the general population today in spite of all our "medical advances." And they even ate lard almost every day. *Lard!*

Their diet should be your diet.

About Processed Foods

Processed food isn't food.

No book about hormones would be complete if you didn't understand something incredible. A study recently published in the *Journal of Applied Toxicology* (March, 2012, pgs. 219-32) showed that thousands of consumer products – processed "foods" – contains hormone-mimicking preservatives!

That means, you are getting hormone therapy every time you eat a box of <fill-in-favorite-junk-food-here>.

And guess what? If you don't need hormone therapy, you certainly shouldn't have it.

The primary culprit is the *paraben* which is often found in processed food preservatives at a rate of *one million times higher than estrogen levels found in human breasts*. These parabens mimic estrogen hormones. And the parabens are found in food, drugs, and cosmetics.

The reason women tend to have more fat than men is because women have over 1,000 times the concentration of estrogen receptors that men have. Our world constantly floods our bodies with estrogen and these parabens that mimic estrogen. But if you're a woman and are afraid of excess estrogens in your body, consider what it does to your husband or boyfriend who were designed to have far less estrogen levels than you. And more frightening, consider what the environment's excess estrogen does to your children!

A wide range of Erectile Dysfunction drugs are sold now for men. A vast number of breast cancers are found in both women *and* men. Children are reaching puberty at ages as young as eight years old. Hormones are powerful and can be good or bad depending on their quantities. Estrogen is an especially insidious hormone these days given how rampant it is in the environment, in preservatives, in cosmetics, in drugs, and in soy.

If knowing this keeps you from picking up the next box of <fill-in-your-favorite-food-here> the next time you go grocery shopping and forces you to run instead to your organic produce section, then we've done our job.

> **Note:** By the way, good food, real food, food that is good for your hormones and body, is not boring or bland food! Those who understand how to eat well for the brain, hormones, and body also understand the importance of spices. Spices are the underutilized secret of good food *and nutrition* as we explained in *Brain Controlled Weight Loss*. There is a reason why history books are filled with centuries of explorers and pirates hunting for the best spice routes in the medieval world. It's because only recently with the prevalence of processed, pre-packed non-"food" have we forgotten what makes food taste good. Spices make food taste good. Not the hormone-mimicking preservatives and dangerous High Fructose Corn Syrup that forms the foundation of almost everything eaten by today's typical consumer.

Hormonal Enemy #1: Sugar and Sugar Equivalents

Although we could go through every hormone and explain why sugar harms that hormone, it makes far more sense to cover it now in one spot.

The Most Wanted on the hormonal enemy list is sugar.

Name any sugar equivalent and it's just as dangerous: Honey, cane sugar, molasses, High Fructose Corn Syrup, fructose, dextrose, and virtually anything-*ose* actually.

"But didn't our great grandparents eat honey, molasses, fruit, and sugar?" you ask. That is a great question. Yes they did. They even spiked an iced tea with a spoonful of white sugar I bet. Maybe both at lunch *and* dinner!

But they didn't consume *22 teaspoons of sugar a day* and that is what the average American adult eats in one form or another. It gets worse. The average American teenager consumes *34 teaspoons of sugar each and every day* according to the American Heart Association.

That quantity of sugar is unnatural and our bodies simply don't know what to do with it all. The sugar is all around us in everything we eat. And it's worse now than ever. After the McGovern Committee in the 1970s convinced the FDA that fat caused us to get fatter (all evidence is to the contrary in every scientific study ever performed), the low-fat and no-fat products have ballooned in every store. But the fat they removed, the fat that did not make us fat, tasted good. So they had to switch to something that tasted good. So they added sugar.

A lot of sugar.

And over time the food companies, with the full approval of the governmental regulators who are supposed to oversee them instead of enable them, got wise to the fact that Americans realized sugar is deadly so they started putting other forms of sugar in our food to fool us. They called it something else. They used names that didn't have the word "sugar" in them. Like corn syrup. Corn starch. Fructose. High Fructose Corn Syrup. Dextrose.

> **Note:** High Fructose Corn Syrup is corn starch boiled in acid. Its production is cheaper than normal, processed, white sugar but it is worse for you than sugar no matter how many millions of dollars the HFCS industry spends on damage control advertisements on television.

And over time, some Americans realized that all those non-"sugar" sugars still meant sugar so the food companies began reducing the amount of each one of those in our products for the few consumers who read the labels. You don't find one of those sugar equivalents in the first two or three ingredients any longer as much as you used to. But there are multiple *forms* of sugar throughout those ingredients, scattered here and there, so the total quantity of the sugar is still massive even though not one of the sugars gets top billing any longer in the ingredients.

Fooled us again, didn't they?

And we keep getting fatter. Wonder why? And we keep getting more diabetes problems. Wonder why? And we keep getting hypertension, thyroid problems, cholesterol problems. Wonder why?

And we keep getting sold more and more drugs to mask the symptoms that our sugar-laced food gives us. Wonder why the FDA, the Food & *Drug* Administration, never seems to mind?

It cannot be stressed enough: sugar kills. Yes, you can eat sugar in moderation. You know that is not what we're talking about here. We're not talking about moderation; we're talking about overdosing as almost every American does daily.

The number one way to feel better is to stop the sugar overdosing. *Now.* Don't plan to stop it next week. Stop it... *Now.* Don't plan to stop it after you finish the last piece of cake tonight for dessert. Stop it... *Now.*

The number one way to begin aligning your hormones for health is to stop overdosing sugar... *Now.*

The "Good" Sugars: Honey, Molasses, Maple Syrup, Fruit, & Starches

Honey is sugar.

Molasses is sugar.

Maple syrup is sugar.

Fruit is sugar.

If you get only organic honey, molasses, maple syrup, and fruit, guess what? They are all sugar also and the damage done is the same.

Organic sugar isn't better for you than other sugar. It just isn't *quite* as deadly as the non-organic sugar. Sort of like a .40 caliber bullet isn't *quite* as deadly as a .45 caliber bullet.

Should you stop eating all those more natural sugar items? Re-read the previous section about the damage that sugar does to your body and hormones and consider this: To play it safe, you should stop honey, molasses, maple syrup, and even fruit at least for a while until you can wean your body off sugar.

> **Note:** If you want an easy and cheap way to get sugar out of your diet while losing weight and improving your hormones, go read Jennifer's *1 Day Diet* book.

If you don't consider yourself a sugar, candy, or dessert person, there is still a huge chance you're addicted to sugar if you're an average American due to the amount of sugar you get elsewhere like in bread and pasta. And if you're not an American reading this, guess what? The reason your nation's thyroid problems, diabetes problems, cancer, and heart maladies have increased dramatically is that your nation isn't too far behind America in its injection of some form of sugar into virtually everything you eat.

Bread, corn, and potatoes are not sugar. However, starchy simple carbohydrates break down almost instantly into sugar as far as your body is concerned.

For most people reading this book, you need to be eating far less bread even if you don't eat desserts in traditional forms. Go *right now* and grab that loaf of bread on your counter, even if it's some fancy-named *High Heavy Multi-Grain Nut Stone-Milled* bread. Look at its ingredients. Go ahead, we'll wait here... Did you see it? The odds are great that your "healthy" bread has HFCS (High Fructose Corn Syrup). Look again if you didn't see it. It's rare that a loaf of bread sold today does not have HFCS.

No wonder you don't eat dessert. You don't have to! You get dessert every time you have a piece of toast, twice with every sandwich, once with every bowl of soup, and once with your salad from the eight croutons on top (not to mention the amount of sugar in the fat-free salad dressing).

Getting back to honey, every health food nut says honey is great for us, right? Honey is sugar. If sugar is bad, honey is bad.

Can honey help with allergies? Yes it can! If you can find an organic honey supplier within a few miles from your home, eating that honey may help your allergies and perhaps boost your immune system. Buying any other honey does not. And buying almost any honey sold on a supermarket shelf isn't even honey but is Chinese-supplied substitute that looks and feels like honey but is just a thick sugar slime.

If you find an organic honey supplier within a few miles of your home, keep that honey in your family's dietary mix. Half a teaspoon or perhaps a whole teaspoon every few days should be the limit. Anything more and the damage done by the honey's sugar far offsets any advantage done by the local honey.

You've heard that molasses is good for you, right? It can be! Organic black strap molasses is a great source of potassium. If you can find it (Amazon sells a good one here: http://www.amazon.com/Organic-Blackstrap-Molasses-15-oz/dp/B000QV19BM/ref=sr_1_1?ie=UTF8&qid=133746661 7&sr=8-1) then keep that molasses in your family's dietary mix. Half a teaspoon every few days. Just like the organic honey, anything more and the damage done by the molasses's sugar far offsets any advantage done by the organic black strap molasses.

You've heard that "real" maple syrup can be good for you, right? It can be! If you buy organic Grade B (never even *think* about buying Grade A ever again) Maple Syrup then you'll be getting the real thing, made to be eaten the way nature intends you to eat it. (Amazon sells a good one here: http://www.amazon.com/Coombs-Family-Farms-Organic-32-Ounce/dp/B00271OPVU/ref=sr_1_cc_1?s=aps&ie=UTF8& qid=1337467606&sr=1-1-catcorr.) Keep that organic Grade B maple syrup in your family's dietary mix. (Perhaps you can now predict what you're about to read next!) Half a teaspoon every few days. Anything more and the damage done by the Grade B maple syrup's sugar far offsets any health advantage done by the organic Grade B maple syrup.

Are you beginning to see a pattern?

By the way, why do you really need maple syrup? If you just love the taste then great, have it in the quantities described above. But if you need it for pancakes and waffles, guess what? As a general rule you should never in your life eat pancakes or waffles again. As a general rule. They are far worse than bread. And they are worse than fruit too. And you're about to see why fruit *can* be horrid.

This would be an insane book if it said don't eat fruit, right? This book will never say that. But fructose, the sugar in fruit, is actually *the worst sugar in existence* according to many reliable sources. Want your eyes opened in a way you never thought possible? Watch the following YouTube video about fructose, which is fruit sugar. It's called *Sugar: The Bitter Truth* and is here: http://www.youtube.com/watch?v=dBnniua6-oM&ob=av3e.

Remember those great-grandparents I keep talking about? You know, the ones who had healthy hormones all their lives? Yes, they ate fruit and perhaps a lot of it. They ate the fruit they grew. The fruit with its skin. When they had juice they would squeeze a couple of oranges or grapefruits once in a while into a glass and a lot of the pulp would fall into the glass too. Also, they'd have it with their morning meal. A meal full of eggs and bacon, often cooked in lard. *Lard!*

It turns out that the way fruit naturally occurs, with its skin (obviously not bananas with their skins; they are extremely high in sugar any way and generally should be reserved as an ultra-rare treat) is the way you should eat it. And it turns out that if you have a meal with lots of fat such as farm-raised, nitrite-free, nitrate-free, bacon made from pigs that led a happy life rooting up the field they were raised in, cooked in lard (*Lard!*) coming from those same happy pigs all slows down the negative effects of real fresh-squeezed fruit juice.

Note: Fat slows down your insulin secretions which is one reason why whole milk causes you to gain less weight than skim milk. The fat slows down the milk sugar known as *lactose.*

So yea. Great-Granny ate fruit and drank her own fruit juice. If you can mimic the way she did it, by picking an apple off your own tree for instance, then go for it. I envy you! But if your source of fruit is your grocer, even if organic, then treat fruit in the future the way you treat dessert and bread today before you read this chapter: eat fruit in moderation, perhaps one serving daily, twice if one or both servings are berries which are low on the glycemic scale and don't affect your blood sugar as negatively as other fruit.

The orange juice in the cans and cartons? You should eat an ice cream sundae instead. Because then you are being honest with yourself. Then you will not be surprised when your hormones get all out of whack as they are going to anyway with all that orange juice over time.

> **Note:** If you really want a sugar substitute, use Stevia and nothing else. Stevia is made from a plant and has zero effect on your glycemic index load. Just about all other artificial sweeteners make you crave sugar and elevate the acidity of your body's pH which increases your chances to get sick. In addition, artificial sweeteners cause water retention and bloating.

Protein and Sugar

Before this book is through you're going to see that a building block of hormones, primarily protein, is extremely vital in your diet. If you've been eating a traditional diet, meaning whatever you see, you've been overloading with carbs and under-loading with healthy fats and good proteins.

When you increase your protein intake, as you'll do if you want to maintain healthy hormones and look great and feel great, the effect of a sugary drink, dessert, or fruit juice from a can or bottle, is exaggerated in your system. Just as fat can slow down effects of sugar somewhat as you'll see in the next section, protein ramps up sugar's effects. So adding protein to your diet is almost always wise to do, but if you maintain your current sweet tooth, the damage done by the sugar will be increased. Don't decrease the protein though; decrease the sugar.

Fat Makes Us Thin

It's true that most dieticians, doctors, FDA regulators, and TV commercials all work hard to convince you that fat in your diet needs to be reduced. To make it real easy, for 30 years the government's Food Pyramid put fat at the very apex of the pyramid, the smallest part of the graphic, to warn you against the dangers of fat.

Gary Taubes wrote an outstanding, but extremely high-level, advanced, scientific volume entitled, "Good Calories, Bad Calories" in which he shows systematically how adding fat back into your diet will systematically force your cells to release fat stores and you'll lose weight. Not one objective government study was ever performed to see how fat affects weight gain or weight loss. But activists on the McGovern Committee that eventually produced the recommendations that led to the government's Food Pyramid said animal fat is bad for us and (surprise) we should not eat meat.

One might be led to think a conspiracy took place.

Good Fat is Good for You

To begin getting your hormones into gear, you need to eat more fat. Fat should be as much as 30 to 35% of your diet with most of the fat coming from animal sources such as grass-fed beef, wild Alaskan salmon (which has low levels of mercury unlike just about any other fish you can get today), farm-raised nitrate-free nitrite-free pork (if you eat pork), free-range chickens, organic seeds, nuts, and healthy oils.

So fats are good? Yes, but not all of them! There is a huge difference between manufactured fats and naturally-occurring healthy fats.

Both the health and food experts such as Gary Taubes *and* the traditional government lackeys such as medical schools agree that trans fats are bad for us. They are bad for us. Trans fats are also called *unsaturated fats*. Stay away from any kind of fat or cooking oil labeled trans fat, unsaturated fat, monosaturated fat, or polysaturated fat. This deadly fat messes with your whole body and never in a good way, from your hormones to your heart to your cholesterol.

Polyunsaturated vegetable oils and fats can become toxic and unstable when heated due to creation of free radicals that damage our cells. Trans fats from hydrogenated oils and margarine are like plastics. They interfere with cells communications between each other, which leads to health dysfunction and chaos at the cell level.

Many fats are great though. Tropical fats are wonderful for us. Cook your family's eggs each morning in organic or extra virgin coconut oil. (We both use extra virgin coconut oil as our main cooking oil for eggs every morning. It contains healthy fat and the lauric acid in them is antimicrobial and fights off bacteria and virus infections.) Make sure you get dark olive oil and always get it in dark, glass bottles because olive oil begins to turn rancid quickly from light. In addition, the lighter-shades of olive oil are indicators of being bleached in peroxide and other solvents and why would you ever want that?

> **Note:** Try organic macadamia nut oil for a nice surprising taste. Ghee is also a wonderful butter.

Speaking of macadamia nuts, organic nuts and seeds are wonderful sources of fats and minerals and vitamins. Make organic nuts and seeds a regular part of your family's diet with a couple of tablespoons of mixed nuts and seeds daily. Did you know that four Brazil nuts each day is all you need to give your body its needed and important selenium? Popping four delicious Brazil nuts is a lot more fun than popping a selenium supplement.

You know all about margarine, right? Now forget everything you know about it. Margarine is a trans fat. Throw it away *now*. If you just bought a new package of anything labeled, "I can't understand why this delicious yellow stuff isn't butter" then throw it away faster than if it was arsenic in your refrigerator! Never use it again.

Buy only organic real butter. Better yet, you can make your own butter from fresh, raw, whole milk (which you can source here: http://www.westonaprice.org/ for raw, whole milk in the states where it's legal to buy it) and make your own butter. You don't need to keep real butter in your fridge by the way. It stays soft outside the fridge.

Avocados are high in good fat. They provide one of the best sources of fat you can find. Eating a half avocado at lunch and at dinner goes a long way toward fulfilling your hormonal need for good fats. By the way, you can store half an avocado in the refrigerator as long as you put it in a baggie and leave the big seed in the half that goes in the fridge.

In summary, a lack of natural fats in your diet makes you gain weight. Natural fats are essential for your cells to work properly. Fats stabilize blood sugar levels, decrease cravings, and make you feel full.

Your Cells and Hormones Love Protein

Throughout the following chapters that cover specific hormones you're going to see a lot of talk about eating more protein. Most hormones are made of protein. That is one reason why low-protein diets such as the Pritikin Diet are so dangerous to your hormonal balance. (The Pritikin Diet is dangerous also due to its strict limitation on fats. If you were to take a drug company's favorite dietary plan for America, it would almost certainly look like the Pritikin Diet. It also looks like the FDA's Food Pyramid.)

You should eat more protein. Something in the neighborhood or 30% of your daily food intake should be good protein.

> **Note:** Good protein never includes soy. Or any ingredient that contains the word "soy" on the label anywhere.

Don't wait for an imbalance of hormones from a blood test. Just start eating more protein. *Now.*

Fix a bunch of organic, cage-free eggs in the morning for you and your family. Cook those eggs in organic, extra virgin coconut or olive oil. Eat up!

Eggs are perhaps the most perfect food in existence. They are literally *life building blocks.* Your hormones will benefit immediately from more eggs in your diet.

And yes, you also need meat. Grass-fed beef, cage-free chicken, mercury-free fish, and free-rooting free-range locally-grown pork.

Note: Nuts are a double-bonus for your hormones, body and weight because they provide both healthy fats and healthy proteins.

A Sidebar About Food

While writing this book, Rich, my co-author was getting tested for heavy metals. Living in the modern world exposes us to all sorts of toxins, both from industrial sites, products used in the building of homes and offices, aluminum from deodorants and old aluminum cookware (you should use an aluminum-free deodorant and only stainless steel and cast iron cookware without exception), mercury (from amalgam fillings and vaccinations and farm-raised fish), and plastics (if you like plastic containers, buy only BPA-free plastic), and municipal water supplies. It's good to be tested every ten years or so to see if you need to detox from those and other toxins that stay in your cells.

Here is his experience: While waiting for the test, I was discussing health issues with an older lady who was there and she told me that she had been to see her parents who are in their 80s living several hundred miles away. Their health has been failing. Her father was overweight and her mother kept telling her, "Your Dad eats and eats, crackers and baloney sandwiches, and he's never full, he's always hungry!"

This lady, who's extremely health conscious, looked in her parents' cabinets and said, "This is why! You don't eat food. All you eat are substances that are sold in boxes and plastic jugs." She began teaching her Mom and Dad all about real food. She told me that she was surprised because they grew up on a farm and always were healthy and strong but it's like they now get everything in a container and trust the grocery to sell them only things that are good for them.

She was surprised that they lived this long given what was in their kitchen cabinets.

I explained to her that being raised in a natural environment of the farm is why they *are* probably still alive. Their initial formative years of growth and hormonal development were with real food and hard work on the farm. That early health investment probably enabled them to live as long as they have. She is making arrangements to get them to come live with her so she can begin reversing their food plight back to what she kept calling "real food." I have no doubt that to the extent she is able to do so, that her parents' last few years will be better for it.

We want to encourage you to begin eating only "real food" today.

Don't believe the Food Pyramid.

Believe your great grandparents who ate lots of eggs, butter, cooked in lard (*Lard!*), chickens, cattle, bacon, vegetables they grew organically before "organic" was a garden-related word, and perhaps four teaspoons of sugar total daily from good fruit sources with the skin that they grew and an *occasional* sugar cube or honey scoop or maple syrup.

Hundreds of millions of great grandparents can't be wrong.

About Carbohydrates

You need carbs along with your good fats and proteins.

Carbs are not your enemy.

Only some carbs are your enemy.

Plus carbs in large quantities can be your hormone and bodily enemies. Sugar, after all, is a carb. When eating carbs, try to limit your carb intake to about 20% to 25% of your daily food.

These suggested percentages are not fixed and you should not take them religiously. Worrying about your daily mix or fats/proteins/carbs can make you as crazy as counting calories and soon you'll just stop altogether if you fret too much with all the numbers. So eating 35%-40% of your diet in healthy fats, 30-35% in protein, and 20% in carbs and the remaining 10-20% fill in with whatever one of those you happen to have more of that day is a great general strategy. Don't fret the actual numbers.

But in general more fat and more protein and fewer carbohydrates than you eat now is what you should begin focusing on from this point forward. That means from now on, not during a "diet phase" but for a lifelong strategy for healthy hormones, healthy brains, and healthy bodies.

In general, as long as your carbohydrates are comprised of colorful vegetables, you can eat up!

By the way, I don't consider *brown* a color in the category "colorful vegetable." This means potatoes are basically out. For good. Yep, this means French fries and baked potatoes. Sorry, I love French fries too but I haven't eaten them for ages. I don't miss them. If I began eating them I'd begin craving them again. So I know from experience that strong bad cravings go away right after you begin eating healthy and real foods.

Potatoes not only are starchy and have a high glycemic index that spikes your blood sugar and weight gain and hormone imbalance worse than scoop of a full fat ice cream (literally), they also are root vegetables. They receive the bulk of pesticides sprayed on farms and gardens through runoff into the ground water where potatoes sit and grow.

You should eat green, leafy vegetables such as kale, lettuce (the greener the variety the better), spinach, okra, green beans, brown beans, all sorts of colorful peppers (even the hot ones, your metabolism gets a major boost every time!), squash, and tomatoes (technically tomatoes are fruit and amazingly they are *healthier* and more nutritious when cooked unlike most vegetables that should never be cooked too much if at all).

I'll go ahead and say carrots as long as you get a wide array of other vegetables.

Stick to the green and colorful fibrous vegetables and you don't really need to concern yourself with a percentage of how much you eat. Just be sure that you have protein and fat at every meal. In general always eat your vegetables with protein and fat so you're not eating only carbs at any time.

If you like salad, do what the expensive restaurants do and cook slices of cage-free chicken to put over the salad and then sprinkle some walnuts and pecans on the salad. What a perfect combination! You'll get full from the salad, your short-term energy levels will be high due to the colorful veggies, and your long-term energy levels will remain high due to the chicken and nut proteins, and you won't feel full until it's truly time to eat next.

Note: You may not believe us until you try it but here it goes: get some organic, extra-virgin olive oil, such as this bottle by the wonderful company Bragg: http://www.amazon.com/Bragg-Organic-Extra-Virgin-Olive/dp/B0006Z7NPO/ref=sr_1_1?ie=UTF8&qid=133 7472219&sr=8-1 and then stop using all salad dressing that you don't make yourself. First, sprinkle *only* olive oil on your salad, use enough to wet your salad adequately, and take a taste. You expect something bland and boring, right? It's not. People often do the vinegar and oil mix, and we like that okay, but just the olive oil makes a surprisingly tasty salad! Plus, the olive oil gives you more of that wonderful healthy fat that your hormones love.

Grains Are Basically Bad

A little bread can be nice can't it?

"Our daily bread" is often a comfort food. By now you're no doubt convinced we're going to talk you out of buying most bread at most stores. True!

But don't toss the baby out with the bath water.

Know that, the best bread is bread that you or a friend makes from fresh, organic, ground wheat. You can get organic wheat to grind into bread in large "superpails" that stay good up to 15 years from Walton Feed (http://waltonfeed.com/). Make sure you make "heavy" bread, bread with seeds and nuts in it. The grain will add fiber to your diet and the seeds and nuts will add to the taste and add protein and fat to the bread which slows down the negative effects of the bread's carbohydrate impact on your body.

Still, you don't want to over-eat this "good" bread. A slice or *maybe* two daily is the very outside maximum you should eat. Your body was not designed to handle many grains and you eat far too much bread right now if you're like the average person.

> **Note:** To help eliminate the negative effects of bread, you can add homemade or store-bought organic butter and extra virgin olive oil. To do as the Romans do, ground some organic, black pepper on top of all that oil and butter that you dribble all over the slice. The fat in the oil and butter does two things: makes the bread taste about as good as anything *can* taste and the bread will then have less impact on your blood sugar making the bread harder to show on your thighs! This is why a white, plain bagel clocks in at a higher glycemic load (meaning it impacts your blood sugar more and makes you fatter) than a scoop of premium ice cream! And low-fat yogurt almost doubles the glycemic load of that premium ice cream. Fat not only does *not* make you fat but it helps reduce the impact of food on your body. That's great because it tastes great and, for our purposes here, fat also is good for your hormones!

Remember that the Food Pyramid put grains on the very bottom layer. That's the thick, largest section. The FDA wants you to make the largest part of your diet breads and grains and (ugh!) cereals. (Cereals are the worst! What's worse than a starchy grain-based carb? A *processed, sugary* starchy grain-based carb!) Since the FDA put grains on the bottom, you can be assured they are the unhealthiest part of the diagram. Always turn the Food Pyramid upside down. Make grains the smallest portion of your daily diet.

Stack Your Food Advantages

We hear from the oatmeal lovers sometimes who despair they must give up their beloved morning grain. Do you love oatmeal and cannot see yourself giving it up altogether? Okay. Then stack your advantages to get the fiber and protein from the oatmeal by doing this: From Walton Feed buy a bucket of organic *oat groats*. Oatmeal is made from a special form of oats called oat groats. A bucket should last your family for a year or so. Get a grinder that has an oat press attachment.

When you or your family want oatmeal, put a couple of scoops of oat groats in your grinder and turn the handle a few turns. Out comes oatmeal. If you taste it, you will taste... oatmeal! Only it will be different from the processed and dead oats you get in the tall cardboard cylinders from the processed food aisle at your grocery store because these oats will have a rich taste you never knew was possible. Plus, you have about an hour before the nutrients inside that pressed, rolled oat go dormant. Feed your family that oatmeal, perhaps as a special treat, or at most in small dishes to accompany a healthy breakfast with eggs and meat, and you will be eating *healthy* oatmeal perhaps for the first time in your entire life. Just don't overdo it. Your body can't process a lot of grains or carbs well.

The idea is always to stack your food advantages. If you want oatmeal then eat it fresh-ground. That way you get the vitamins and minerals. Never eat refined grains which are most of the grains eaten today. Refining grains removes fiber which is the healthiest part of the grain and affects your digestion. If you normally eat anything with grains that says "fortified with..." throw it away *now* and never buy it again. The reason food processors have to fortify food is because the real food has been turned into dead food that has to be revamped so the label can say it's a source of vitamins. It's easier, and tastes far better as you'll see with oatmeal made from fresh-rolled oat groats, if you stick with real food to begin with and not eat anything in a package.

Driving through Kansas recently, I saw miles and miles of corn fields. It's easy to forget that corn is not a vegetable but it's a grain. Like any grain, you want to limit corn in your family's diets. Your hormones react to corn about the same way they react to sugar because corn is a simple carbohydrate that becomes sugar quickly to your body.

Corn is worse than you might imagine. If you ever get a chance to see the documentary *King Corn* you should. You'll never eat the stuff again. Now while that would be fine, fresh, organic corn can certainly be a tasty and *rare* treat. What you may not know though is that corn is in everything you probably have eaten to this point. It's in almost every processed food. It's in almost every sugar equivalent. It's in all the non-diet soda you have drank the past couple of decades. (Diet soda is no better and is often worse with its aspartame and other chemical, phony sweeteners.)

> **Note:** You can get the movie *King Corn* here in DVD format: http://www.amazon.com/King-Corn-Standard-Packaging-Bledsoe/dp/B001EP8EOY/ref=sr_1_2?ie=UTF8&qid=1337473841&sr=8-2 and it's cheap! Even better, at the time of this writing, Amazon Prime members can watch the streaming version of *King Corn* for free here: http://www.amazon.com/King-

Corn/dp/B003F9XQ9A/ref=tmm_aiv_title_0?ie=UTF8&
qid=1337473841&sr=8-2.

Corn is also in almost every bite of meat you eat!

From cradle to grave, most cattle, chickens and pigs are raised on a steady diet of corn. They are what they ate! This transfers to your system. Instead of grass for the cattle and bugs for the chickens and slop for the pigs they eat nothing... but... corn.

Then you get it second-hand. Like second-hand smoke, second-hand corn is bad for you and your hormones and your body. It's no longer "real" beef when the beef you eat was raised on a grain that its system was never designed to eat.

> **Note:** Fish farms feed fish a steady diet of soy. So when you eat most fish, especially any and all that comes in a package or canned, you're getting second-hand soy.

The next time you get a hankering for corn, keep all of this in mind. You probably already had more than your share of corn today second-hand. Until your diet consists of real food and real meat raised properly, you should avoid all corn.

Salt is Not Demonic

Salt is one of the most maligned foods of the past 50 years and is far less deadly than it's been blamed for in most people. Generally, someone who eats a diet rich in animal protein and healthy fats will not have a salt imbalance. Actually, you may find that you need to *add* salt to get enough of it. Let your cravings be your guide. But as you cease eating phony food from packages you will naturally get less salt and your body needs salt to perform well.

Still, a high craving for salt can result in a salt/potassium imbalance that does eventually cause you problems. A repaired serotonin level can help repair your salt craving and help return your sodium/potassium levels back to where they should be: in balance.

Some heart patients need to reduce salt. But salt is not bad for your heart in general and for a healthy society we need to look at some truth behind this condiment that is a required part of a healthy diet.

Like red meat, fat, and the sun, salt has gotten a tremendously bad rap. Your body needs an ample supply of sodium to function properly. When you begin to eat better you will eat fewer sugary or fast foods because your brain will want fewer of those kinds of things. Your sodium intake will go from a high amount of bad, processed, white salt to not enough salt.

Get salt and use it! Make sure, however, it is *sea salt*. Don't be afraid of it, especially as you eat higher quality foods that won't have as much sodium as the foods you used to binge on. I always carry either Celtic brand or Real Salt brand with me. Of the two, my preference is for the Real Salt brand. You can get it on Amazon.com here: http://www.amazon.com/Real-Salt-Sea-Pouch-26-Ounce/dp/B000BD0SDU/ref=sr_1_1?ie=UTF8&qid=1337473780&sr=8-1.

We only let our families eat "sea salt." Sea salt is unprocessed (if you buy a good brand) and doesn't look uniformly white and is not as uniformly ground as the white, processed garbage you've seen. That is good and you should expect it. You will also find that it tastes much better than the typical salt. It's also much healthier for your body and hormonal balance than traditional table salt.

Sea salt has 84 different minerals whereas the typical table salt has only two.

Balance Your Fats, Proteins, and Carbs

"Everything in moderation" is good hormonal and health advice *if* you have your basic diet correct. That is, eating healthy fats, healthy protein, and limiting your carbohydrates to leafy, fibrous, colorful vegetables, moderate your fruit intake emphasizing berries and treating other fruit like you may have treated dessert before this book, and virtually eliminating all sugar and equivalents and eat hearty bread in extreme moderation such as one slice daily.

If you over-emphasize any of the three food divisions your hormones will suffer. For example, if you eat 50% or more of your diet in fat, even if you limit yourself to healthy animal and tropical fats, your HGH (Human Growth Hormone) will begin to shut down. If you eat too much protein, such as 50% or more, your thyroid hormone can mess up your metabolism as well as lots of other things. Eating 25% or more of your diet in carbs, especially starchy carbs and desserts, is going to overload your body with sugar, add weight, and affect your insulin negatively.

So you are to eat more fat, eat more protein, eat fewer carbs, but if you eat too much fat, too much protein, or too many carbs and you'll mess everything up at the hormonal level! This can drive us crazy, right? The answer is simple. At every meal make sure you eat good fats, good protein, and a side of fibrous veggies. The numbers will take care of themselves and so will your hormones. Don't fret over the numbers. Turn the FDA's Food Pyramid upside down, emphasize the food types on the new bottom layers, stay away from sugar, starches, and grains as much as possible, and you'll stay balanced.

More About that Sugar

Can you eliminate all non-fruit sweets from your life for a while? If there is any way you can do that you *will* stop craving sugar. At first your body is going to go into minor withdrawals meaning you might crave sugar quite a bit and perhaps even feel shaky the first day or two depending on how much you eat now. That doesn't last long.

Our bodies secrete the hormone insulin to metabolize the food we eat. That is normal and that is what we want. The problem is that our bodies secrete insulin in much higher amounts when the foods are high in sugar or when our overall diets are high in bad carbs. Sugar damages your tissues so that your body tries to expel it from the bloodstream. We'll discuss problems with sugar and bad carbs more when we get to the hormones affected most.

Higher insulin amounts make you feel hungrier and you end up eating more. That is why so many restaurants bring you a basket of bread before taking your order. That is also why Mexican restaurants bring you a basket of chips faster than Speedy Gonzales before giving you a menu. That high-carb, low-fat, low-fiber bread and those chips spark your insulin secretion, lowers your body's ability to metabolize food, and makes you want to eat far more than you would have *before* filling up on bread.

Are you beginning to see the food-hormone connection?

Now for the Hormones

With the basic hormone-balancing diet out of the way, you need to focus now on specific hormones. By learning about the key hormones that affect your health and weight, you will learn to spot problems when they develop and learn ways to emphasize or use diet to augment specific hormones when an imbalance occurs.

CHAPTER 5

THE MASTER CONTROL HORMONE

–

THYROID HORMONE

As with all the hormones we discuss in this book, we're not out to make you a scientist. The truth is that hormones can be a complex subject. Why complicate things? You want to be healthy and be at an optimum weight. That's our focus here.

It should be no surprise that your thyroid gland produces the thyroid hormone. The thyroid gland is located at the bottom of the front part of your neck.

Actually, there are two thyroid hormones: thyroxine and triiodothyronine. Fortunately they are also referred to by the easier names of T4 and T3. T4 forms the bulk of your thyroid ` hormone group with the most active part being T3. For the purposes of this book, we'll just call T4 and T3 the thyroid hormone and consider them as a pair to be a single group.

Your thyroid gland has a major job: it controls your metabolism (among other things including your energy levels). For someone interested in weight loss, therefore, getting the thyroid in balance is vital.

Problems with Thyroid Imbalance

"It's a glandular problem."

That is what people used to say about overweight people who couldn't seem to lose weight. It would often be said politely to help excuse the weight. It might be said sarcastically to mock the obese person. It may be said of the overweight person herself to try to mask or get needed sympathy for her plight (or his).

The thing is, being overweight *is* a glandular problem. Fortunately, it can be corrected in almost all cases. If you are overweight, it's almost a sure sign that your thyroid gland is not producing proper thyroid hormone levels.

Another sign of thyroid problems is not just weight gain but swelling in the ankles and fingers can also be a sign of potential thyroid problems. These are symptoms of the thyroid hormone trouble but also portend other problems such as low energy levels. It takes more energy to drag excess weight, and even swollen fingers and other body parts can make you sluggish.

Your fatigue from a thyroid imbalance adds to your weight gain in other ways too. With fatigue comes a false signal of hunger. This fatigue-related hunger signal usually makes you crave what is commonly called "comfort food." Traditionally comfort food is all the bad stuff: mashed potatoes, gravy, bread, corn, cake, and ice cream. By eating those heavy and bad carbs your thyroid goes into meltdown even further! It's a high-carb lifestyle that messes up a lot of thyroid problems to begin with.

Chronic fatigue syndrome, a problem that was almost unheard of just a decade ago, has been on the rise. Thyroid imbalances causes that fatigue. This results in increased depression.

Your thyroid also can produce non-metabolism related problems such as:

- Hair loss

- Dry and brittle hair and nails

- Extreme sensitivity to cold in your hands and feet

- Muscle and joint aches

- Low sex drive

- Menstrual cycle maladies

- Gastronomical problems such as constipation

- Lowered thinking ability

Thyroid issues have caused the drug industry to substantially boost its pills and liquids to treat the symptoms including an increased use of antidepressants, menstrual drugs, energy pills and drinks, pain relievers, sex drive boosters, laxatives, gelatin tablets, and so on.

Wouldn't it be easier and cheaper to treat the cause (the thyroid) and not all the symptoms? You can and the best news is that you often can treat the cause with diet alone.

Hypothyroidism

Fatigue-related thyroid problems are grouped together into a category known as *hypothyroidism*. Hypothyroidism is the result of an under-active thyroid that produces too few thyroid hormones. Hypothyroidism, therefore, is a deficiency in thyroid hormones. You can exercise all day but you just won't lose weight or keep it off. Your body won't allow that. There is not enough thyroid activity to metabolize the fat.

As I discuss in my book, *Hypothyroidism Diet Tips & Tricks for Women – Fix Your Thyroid & Lose Weight Fast*, Women are especially prone to hypothyroidism and get hypothyroidism almost ten-to-one over men. The most common age range is in the 40s where hypothyroidism flares up.

By moving less because you feel so tired, you don't get the daily benefit of normal caloric burning through movement as much as you would if you were more active.

Hyperthyroidism

Your thyroid doesn't just cause problems by being sluggish.

The opposite of hypothyroidism is *hyperthyroidism*. That is when your thyroid goes into hyper-activity. At first you might think hyperthyroidism is beneficial because if hypothyroidism makes you gain weight, then shouldn't we all strive for hyperthyroidism?

No, not at all.

We should all strive for a balanced thyroid. We want our thyroid hormone group to be at its optimum level the way they were designed to be.

The autoimmune disease known as *Graves Disease* is a type of hyperthyroidism. Fortunately, only a small number of people are susceptible to hyperthyroidism, around 2% for women and only about 0.2% of men. Excess sweating, hypersensitivity to heat, severe weight loss, and diarrhea can be present in hyperthyroidism's symptoms. You might note these are almost the mirror-image of hypothyroidism's symptoms of being cold all the time, weight gain, and constipation.

You want neither hyperthyroidism not hypothyroidism.

Putting Your Thyroid in Balance

Those with thyroid problems have several non-medical tips to try and many people see good results without going the drug route.

First, iodine supplementation is often suggested as a means to bring your thyroid into balance. Next to a deficiency in vitamin D3, nutritionists are beginning to suspect that a lack of iodine in our diets contributes to problems never-before seen in the numbers we see them today. Decades and decades ago the RDA (*recommended daily allowance*) of nutrients was designed and has hardly been updated since.

So our RDA of nutrients such as iodine has not increased but the problem is that the food we eat *has* decreased in the nutrients we get from it. So whereas out great grandparents might have done well on a "normal" diet back then, today's "normal" is anything but normal when it comes to healthy bodies and balanced hormone. The RDA for iodine has been said to be off as much as an *entire decimal place*, meaning instead of the 10 or so mcg (micrograms) suggested, we need as much as 10 to 15 mgs (milligrams) daily... about 100 times the RDA's suggested level.

A blood test can tell you immediately how your thyroid health is doing. But if your thyroid is out of balance, certainly you owe it to yourself to try some iodine supplementation and better food before you go the thyroid medicine route. Let your nutritionist determine from your blood test what levels of iodine you should supplement with, if any. Excess levels of iodine are just as bad as low levels. Excess iodine blocks the enzymes that produce thyroid hormones.

You might think you get ample supplies of iodine in salt. It's true that salt *can* be beneficial to your thyroids health. Still, salt as it is generally eaten is not good for you. It is processed and the iodine is a mass-produced substance that, like most "enriched" food and condiments, has better alternatives. Instead of the perfectly-symmetrical table salt, start using only sea salt as discussed earlier in this book. Sea salt does have traces of iodine but a blood test will tell you if you might need an extra boost in iodine. If so, *Idoral,* a potassium and iodine supplement is available here: http://www.amazon.com/Iodoral-Potency-Potassium-Supplement-Tablets/dp/B000WG3FU4/ref=sr_1_1?ie=UTF8&qid=13375 57425&sr=8-1.

Idoral is a non-prescription supplement and it's great. But as you know, when you can fix or begin to repair any malady with real food, that's always the best alternative. Our problem is that we usually create problems by not eating real food. Polyunsaturated oils like soybean and corn oil block absorption of the iodine needed to make proper levels of the thyroid hormone.

One way to help hypothyroidism is with Brazil nuts. Brazil nuts are high in selenium and selenium helps regulate your thyroid hormones. (Selenium deficiency has been linked to cancer by one study known as the *NPC* and in case that link is proved valid there's another reason to grab those Brazil nuts.) The advantage of eating four or so organic Brazil nuts daily is that you also get some good fat and protein too.

In addition to Brazil nuts, the entire hormone-balanced dietary lifestyle discussed in the previous chapter is almost a perfect food-based prescription for good thyroid balance. All the good fats, the seeds, nuts, and oils, all contribute to help balance your thyroid hormones. (Thyroids especially like cod liver oil by the way even if we don't. Fortunately, cod liver oil is now sold in easy-to-take capsules, such as here: http://www.amazon.com/Barleans-Organic-Oils-Softgels-250-Count/dp/B0031ESWZW/ref=sr_1_6?s=hpc&ie=UTF8&qid =1337558139&sr=1-6)

Quality sourced beef, lamb, and mercury-free fish such as wild Alaskan salmon are great for your thyroid. Vegetables and small amounts of fruit also contribute to thyroid health.

It's been found that snacking between meals not only affects your weight gain but also eating more frequently slows down your thyroid function. Stick to "three square" meals a day. Stay away from sodas, especially diet sodas. Just about any "low-fat" or "no-fat" food labeled as such is phony food that will not help your thyroid at all.

So the next time you sit down to eat a meal, make every bite count and stack all your advantages. Eating a high fat, high protein, low carb, healthy meal with organic produce is going to rev up your master control hormone into superhero gear.

CHAPTER 6

THE FAT-STORING HORMONE

–

INSULIN

Insulin is a hormone produced by your pancreas.

The pancreas shares some space with your stomach by resting right behind it. Its location is perfect because insulin produced by your pancreas gland goes into action when food is present in your system. The type of food you eat determines how much insulin your pancreas produces.

We've already discussed insulin because no book today on health, especially one that is stressing weight loss, could be written honestly without talking about this critical weight-related hormone.

Insulin determines the way our body uses or stores food. Insulin's role is to regulate the metabolism of these two food groups:

- Fat

- Carbohydrates

Diabetes problems have been on the rise ever since the government told everybody how much healthier it is to eat fewer fats and more carbohydrates. Insulin problems are diabetes problems.

How important is insulin? People who live long lives all have normal insulin levels. As you can see, insulin is critical indeed.

A Little Insulin Background

To discuss insulin properly, we must get into the chemical behavior of insulin just a bit more than most of the other hormones.

As we eat carbohydrates, our bodies convert those carbs into sugar which secretes into our bloodstream from our intestines. This is normal and proper. What is improper is when our sugar levels get out of balance which happens as we eat more sugar and fewer fats and proteins.

> **Note:** Even leafy, fibrous vegetables convert to some sugar which is what the glycemic index is all about. The higher the glycemic level a food registers the more impact that food has on your blood sugar. Ultimately, too much blood sugar causes you to store fat. Or worse, get sick.

Sugar, in the form of glucose, is what travels from our intestines to our blood supply. Too much glucose sugar and we die because an abundance of glucose is toxic to us. Our pancreas creates insulin to regulate the amount of glucose in our system. Glucose levels rise while we eat carbs, our pancreas creates more insulin and the insulin is the signal to our liver and muscles and fat tissue to remove glucose from our bloodstream. That removed glucose converts to glycogen and stored in our cells.

The more sugar our food has, the more that glucose rises. Excess insulin causes excess glucose to be removed. As long as everything is in balance, all is well. We can even eat a sweet orange as a treat and the pancreas generates insulin to remove the excess glucose from our blood. The excess glucose can get stored as glycogen and we gain a little weight when that happens.

If we haven't eaten for a while, or if we eat non-sugary foods, our blood glucose levels fall below normal. That is when our bodies begin to use its stored glycogen as energy. The upshot is that we lose some weight every time stored glycogen is used for fuel instead of glucose.

So, although we use sugar for fuel, sugar is damaging to our cell tissues which is why a healthy body performs a constant give-and-take with insulin. A healthy body with a healthy diet works to use carbohydrates for fuel and not for storing fat in cells.

Type 1 Diabetes

Things happen where we don't always produce enough insulin when it's needed.

People with type 1 diabetes don't produce enough insulin. Their bodies enter into a starvation cycle even when they eat because their cells don't utilize the calories from the glucose they pull from their bloodstream. The patients get sick if they don't get regular insulin injections to allow the cells to utilize the glucose properly.

Type 2 Diabetes

Type 2 diabetes is about 9.5 times more common than type 1 diabetes.

Whereas type 1 diabetes patients don't create enough insulin, type 2 diabetes patients often produce too much insulin and the body becomes insulin resistant. The cells ignore insulin signals and don't pull glucose from the bloodstream. Too much glucose in the blood is toxic and type 2 diabetes patients get sick from the high levels of glucose in their blood.

In the past, type 2 diabetes occurred generally in patients in their 40s and older. It even had the label, "adult onset diabetes" that hasn't been used lately due to the new prevalence of the disease in children.

Type 2 diabetes often results from a combination of a genetic predisposition and being overweight. The combination of excess weight and genetics is cause for concern for anyone whose relatives fall into either of those two categories but who have not yet experienced type 2 diabetes problems. Often, a proper diet can counteract the impact of bad genetics.

Problems with Insulin Imbalance

Too little insulin, even in patients who do not have actual type 1 diabetes, can result in these problems:

- Underweight

- Excess urination and bladder pressure due to increased thirst

- Breathing problems dizziness

Too much insulin, even in patients who do not have actual type 2 diabetes, can result in these problems which often are the mirror-images of type 1 diabetes:

- Obesity (obesity can also be part of the cause of type 2 diabetes)

- Menstrual abnormalities

- Depression and fatigue

- Low sex drives

If you are diagnosed with either type 1 or type 2 diabetes, you are probably going to require medical treatment to some degree or another for a long time and perhaps your entire life. Fortunately, many find that diet can help balance the insulin production and diabetes patients have found that proper diets can help reduce the negative effects and the severity of the disease.

Here is a good spot to mention that my *1 Day Diet* book helps to reverse and correct type 2 diabetes by making your body more insulin sensitive. If want to lose weight as fast as possible from a diet (and or you have type 2 diabetes), go check it out.

Putting Your Insulin in Balance

Obviously, if you're diagnosed with diabetes, seek medical help.

Although we're convinced that our bodies are designed to utilize real food to regulate and repair our systems, if we get too far out of balance we require medical help. Not enough time is available to wait on our bodies to fix things if the damage has gone too far.

Note: Insulin affects the production of other hormones including glucagon, leptin, cortisol, testosterone, and estrogen. This is yet another reason to focus on your insulin balance.

For example, if you're diagnosed with type 1 diabetes you must be treated with insulin, either through injections or pumps. Your body requires the insulin for properly digesting all the food you eat. If you're diagnosed with type 2 diabetes, you may be put on medicine depending on the severity but your doctor is going to give you the same advice we will: your diet will have a dramatic impact on how much your type 2 diabetes is a problem in your life.

If your doctor recommends a high carb diet, you'd better get a second opinion. Neither Jen nor Rich are doctors and we don't play one in the books we write. Nevertheless, the more carbs you eat the higher your blood sugar levels will spike. Even a medical doctor trained at the Shrine of the Government Food Pyramid has to agree to that.

Alcohol, starchy foods, and desserts contribute to insulin problems. Just about anything that comes in a box at your grocery store is either a dead food that is neutral or a substance that is going to affect your insulin hormones negatively.

The Role that Exercise Plays

A sedentary lifestyle without exercise can also raise diabetes complications. You don't have to become an exercise guru to escape a sedentary lifestyle. Just get up every hour and walk around if nothing else! Your body is designed for regular activity and that activity doesn't have to be extreme.

Don't try to set exercise time records!

One thing to avoid if you want balanced hormones is extended exercise over weeks and months. When you exercise using a paced, high-intensity followed by low-intensity pattern, your hormones are made healthier and more plentiful when needed. If, however, you are a marathon kind of runner, swimmer, aerobic-related exerciser or you lift weights using set after set 5 days a week or more, your hormones are so busy trying to repair damage done by the exercising that they don't get enough time to regulate your digestive activities.

According to Eric Berg, DC, fat-burning hormones do their best work during resting activities and not exercising activities. Give your body plenty of time to rest and recover from the exercise you choose.

Exercise lowers your insulin levels (and increases glucagon which is win-win for you!). Some diabetes patients monitor their blood sugar levels close to bedtime and if they are too high they must walk on a treadmill or do other forms of exercise until their blood sugar level is low enough to go to sleep safely. Why not get started before you have to lower your blood sugar level before bed every night on a treadmill?

Exercise *tomorrow* if it's dark outside as you read this and exercise *today* if it's still light outside.

Don't *plan* to start exercising, just *start* exercising.

If you have not exercised in a long time just walk in place while you watch television tonight instead of just sitting or lying there. Getting started is the hardest part, so stop *planning* to start and just start. And again, don't believe the aerobics lie that long exercise sessions, such as long-distance running, are healthy. That kind of exercise creates more dangerous free radicals in your body and causes numerous hormonal imbalances over the long term.

Exercise in short, explosive bursts… you'll be challenging your body with what it needs most.

Back to Food

Guess what kind of eating affects insulin problems in a productive, positive way? You guessed it, the healthy hormonal diet discussed in Chapter 4.

The lifestyle comprised of healthy fats, healthy proteins, and a few non-starchy carbs is one of the best ways to regulate your insulin production as much as you can through natural means.

> **Note:** As a general rule, if you have thyroid problems, lightly cook or steam your vegetables. Raw fibrous veggies sometimes have a natural iodine blocking effect. Although this is not a severe restriction you want to stack every advantage you can. Generally, cooked vegetables have fewer nutrients than uncooked but for thyroid problems it's worth losing a *few* nutrients by *lightly* cooking your fibrous greens such as broccoli. As we've said elsewhere, tomatoes actually increase their nutrients and health effects when you cook them lightly.

MSG often found in Asian food and many other items has been shown to *triple* the output of insulin that you produce. Try to avoid any and all Asian food places that don't state they are MSG free.

The supplement called *chromium picolinate* can be an important help for blood sugar regulation. Start with 3,000 mcg (*micro*grams) daily to begin with and reduce that down to 1,000 mcg daily after your sugar cravings go away.

CHAPTER 7

THE FAT-REMOVING HORMONE

–

GLUCAGON

Like insulin, glucagon is a hormone that your pancreas produces.

Glucagon raises low blood sugar when needed. When your blood sugar level gets too low, a healthy pancreas releases glucagon. Glucagon has been called a fat-burning or removing hormone.

You'll recall from the previous chapter that when blood sugar levels get too high, a healthy pancreas releases insulin to remove the glucose from your blood and send that glucose to your other tissue. Isn't the body's regulation system amazing? It's worth balancing your hormones and keeping them balanced because they keep you feeling good through their behind-the-scenes activities such as blood-sugar level regulation.

The bottom line of glucagon is that it melts fat. When your blood sugar levels are low, you'll secrete glucagon so your tissues get needed sugar and energy. Glucagon pulls sugar out of storage, first from the liver, then from fat.

Problems with Glucagon Imbalance

If you have little glucagon, you'll become fat.

If you have too much glucagon, you'll be thinner than you should be.

Although most people dream of being thinner than they should be, such a problem is as dangerous as obesity. Remember that a healthy hormonal balance will not only enable you to lose weight if you're obese but a healthy hormonal balance will add weight if you need that. Your body knows what weight is best for you as long as you focus on your hormones and let them regulate your weight the way they were designed to do.

The way you mess up your glucagon balance is to eat too many bad foods over a long period of time. This is what so many are doing right now. Snacking between meals with a quick candy bar or soda pop also damages glucagon levels.

Note: Pancreatic tumors can be present which almost certainly will lead to out-of-balance glucagon levels so if you have had trouble with weight loss in the past you should have your pancreas checked to make sure it's clear.

If you get hungry between meals, eat a small scoop of organic, mixed nuts. 10 to 20 grams of protein also prevents your body from entering a starvation stage if you go too long without eating. If that happens, your body will begin to crave bad carbs dramatically. Also, your body will try to hang on to fat stores in case the perceived fast lasts a while. Jennifer's *The Ultimate Diet Guide For Busy Women! No Starving, No Food Restrictions, No Gym Workouts Required* tells you the best way to snack to get and maintain a healthy and slim body without adding fat.

Putting Your Glucagon In Balance

When glucagon metabolizes your fat into energy, you lose weight.

Eat natural fats and a good amount of protein while avoiding bad carbs, your insulin secretion is regulated. This also will mean your glucagon is regulated and in order. You'll lose weight. Protein is instrumental in stimulating glucagon.

Exercise also increases glucagon production. You already know that exercise burns fat. But now you know that exercise produces a fat-burning hormone that burns even more fat!

CHAPTER 8

THE "I FEEL-FULL" HORMONE

–

LEPTIN

Leptin is a hormone that controls how full you feel. With no other description you already can see how vital controlling leptin is if you want to control your weight.

Unlike many other hormones, no gland secretes leptin. Your fat cells secrete leptin.

Problems with Leptin Imbalance

Leptin can be a strange hormone in how it gets out of balance.

If you eat too little food you can develop low leptin levels. One problem of calorie-restriction diets – and there are several problems with calorie-restriction diets – is that leptin is reduced. That phenomenon we call "stomach shrinkage" when we eat less over time is not smaller stomachs. The feeling that our stomachs shrink when we eat fewer calories over time is almost certainly lower leptin hormone levels.

In women, menstruation can slow and even stop if leptin hormone levels get too low.

Strict low-carb diets with a restrictive level of all carbohydrates can cause your body to produce too few leptin hormones. The Atkins diet suggests only a few weeks of the "induction phase" which is good because reducing carbs down to 10% or so can drop your leptin levels. This is one reason why some people see how well low-carb diets work and they go overboard without eating enough carbs to maximize their weight loss. In doing so, they damage their leptin levels causing other problems to appear. A balanced diet with all three (fats, proteins, and some carbohydrates) helps ensure your overall health and hormonal balance.

Leptin increases when you eat too many fake, processed foods. You keep eating but your satiety goes into overload and the full switch breaks and you lose control of your appetite. In other words, you keep eating more and more but you never feel full. Leptin levels stop responding properly.

In general, the more you weigh the more leptin you produce. But instead of working for you, the leptin hormone begins working against you. When you are overweight, your leptin hormone level increases but at the same time, that obesity causes those leptin hormones to become sluggish and misfire. In spite of the quantities, they stop turning off your "full" switch. You therefore eat more and more which contributes to the obesity cycle you find yourself on.

Note: Low-fat diets are bad for at least two primary hormones. They lead to both high insulin and high leptin levels.

An article about Dr. Kent Holtorf, MD recently said this in an interview where he linked leptin and thyroid (T3) as key factors in the inability to lose weight:

Dr. Holtorf has discovered that while there are many factors involved in the inability to lose weight, almost all the overweight and obese patients he treats have demonstrable metabolic and endocrinological dysfunctions that contribute to weight challenges. In particular, Dr. Holtorf addresses the evaluation and correction of imbalances in two key hormones – leptin and reverse T3 (rT3) – to help thyroid patients lose weight.

Studies are finding [...] that the majority of overweight individuals who are having difficulty losing weight have varying degrees of leptin resistance, where leptin has a diminished ability to affect the hypothalamus and regulate metabolism. This leptin resistance results in the hypothalamus sensing starvation, so multiple mechanisms are activated to increase fat stores, as the body tries to reverse the perceived state of starvation.

The mechanisms that are activated include diminished TSH secretion, a suppressed T4 to T3 conversion, an increase in reverse T3, an increase in appetite, an increase in insulin resistance and an inhibition of lipolysis (fat breakdown).

These mechanisms may be in part due to a down-regulation of leptin receptors that occurs with a prolonged increase in leptin.

The result? Once you are overweight for an extended period of time, it becomes increasingly difficult to lose weight.

That last sentence is key because it means the longer you go without correcting your leptin and other hormonal balance issues, the harder it is going to be to lose weight. Why not promise yourself *right now* that the next bite you put into your mouth is going to come from a meal with healthy fats, proteins, and fibrous vegetable carbohydrates!

Putting Your Leptin in Balance

To lose weight as quickly as you can you *must* get your leptin into balance.

Healthy fats are crucial for proper leptin balancing. You must maintain your good fats, making them a major part of your lifestyle for the rest of your life. In doing so, you will feel full after eating a good meal and you will feel hungry when you need to eat.

Keep in mind, it is your fat that produces leptin. Leptin, when in balance, tells your brain's hypothalamus that you are full and can stop eating.

Note: Healthy fats and fish contain high levels of something called omega-3 oils which are generally in short supply in the modern, fast food lifestyle. Among other advantages, omega-3 oils boost your feeling of being full after eating and help regulate healthy levels of leptin.

Sleep is critical for proper leptin levels. This means that your sleep hormone – melatonin – also comes into play, indirectly, to regulate leptin.

In addition to healthy fats and more sleep, low leptin levels have been helped by the supplement 5-HTP. 5-HTP, also known as *5-Hydroxytryptophan*, is a by-product of the protein building block called L-tryptophan. You can find a quality 5-HTP supplement here:

http://www.bodybuilding.com/store/now/5htp.html.

CHAPTER 9

THE GROWING UP HEALTHY HORMONE

–

GH/HGH

When little children grow up, they get bigger. They get bigger because they secrete GH – the *growth hormone.*

This GH growth hormone is secreted naturally in your body by your pituitary gland. HGH, or human growth hormone, is created by a fancy technology called *recombinant DNA technology.* In spite of those technical differences most sources, including this one, will refer to HGH and GH interchangeably because the mainstream does so. Unless specifically mentioning a lab-produced growth hormone in which case we'll always stick to the more specific HGH.

HGH affects growth and repair of all your muscles and tissues. The reason the growth hormone can repair your tissues is that it has responsibility for helping to reproduce cells throughout your body. Every one of your body's cells is replaced multiple times as you age. The "you" you started with isn't the same "you" now reading this book!

Therefore you maintain this proper rebuilding of your cells you must maintain a proper level of GH production. You must also maintain a proper weight. Body fat inhibits your production of HGH secretion. If you are overweight then your body is doing everything it can to produce HGH and almost certainly failing.

Problems with HGH Imbalance

The time your body needs high doses of growth hormone is your formative younger years of course. You are growing up and that's why it's called the *growth* hormone. Too much HGH as a child is a rare disorder but can appear once in a while manifesting itself as extra-large (not necessarily overweight) children. Too much as an adult is rare and found mostly in athletes who abuse growth hormone supplements.

As you age, you naturally will produce less HGH. As long as you're otherwise healthy that is fine and even AMA-approved drug-and-cut medical doctors don't prescribe the HGH therapies for patients who are otherwise healthy. So a decrease related to aging is not a major problem. You slow down as you age, your metabolism slows, you eat less, you are less active, your body is expected to do less, so less HGH is often not noticed or a problem. If anything, less growth hormone in an elderly person means that person won't have an over-abundance of HGH which, although rare, can lead to enlargement of bones and breast tissue in men.

Having too little HGH too early is far more common. Children who are far smaller and weaker than other children their age possibly have HGH development problems. Of course diets that make our children fat and diabetic – the government's Food Pyramid-related diets – will put HGH and many other hormones out of balance long before these children have a chance to reach adulthood in a healthy state.

Adults with low HGH production experience several seemingly-unrelated symptoms including:

- Sleep without dreams (routine dreaming is a healthy release for a healthy brain as discussed in our *Brain Controlled Weight Loss*)

- Reduction in overall muscle mass

- Fatigue

- Anxiety

- Lack of sexual interest

- Panic

Sadly, many people and doctors see symptoms such as these and look to psychology and psychiatry to handle them. Out of ignorance and perhaps greed, those fields rarely will do anything to address the hormonal balance issues so many people have today.

Ways to Put Growth Hormone Out of Balance

One way that HGH is kept from being freely produced in your body is through frequent eating. You might be noticing a trend here because other hormones already mentioned such as thyroid production of insulin and glucagon are also negatively affected by frequent eating.

Typically, a weight-loss book will stress that you should eat smaller meals more frequently instead of three large daily. The problem is that this does your hormones no favor. If your hormones become too stressed out working on your digestion functions they won't be putting enough effort into producing balanced hormones. So in general, eating three meals daily is one healthy way to benefit your hormones. When your hormone levels benefit your weight will too as an added bonus. Just be sure to eat plenty of good fat, healthy proteins, and a few fibrous, colorful vegetable carbs with each of those three meals to promote additional hormone balance and weight loss.

> **Note:** HGH levels increase when you fast, but fasting is tricky. Performing a starvation fast for example can wreak havoc with your whole body depending on your condition before you began and how to approach the starvation fast. In addition, starvation fasts are difficult and unnecessary with the good alternatives available if weight is a key goal for you. The *1-Day Diet: The Fastest "Diet" in the World* solves all this fasting mystery for you and is the best diet we know of for weight loss and long-term health.

At the time of this writing, growth hormones cannot be added to cows for beef production or to chickens or pigs. (It's not from a major lack of trying by the largest conglomerate farming producers.) It is still legal to put growth hormones in dairy cows, however, to increase their production of milk.

> **Note:** If you don't yet drink raw, whole milk then why not? Still, if you buy your milk in a carton, skip any milk labeled *bovine somatotropin* because that milk came from growth hormone-injected cows. The long-term effects of such injections passed along to humans is extremely

controversial. Although milk sold as "organic" won't contain the bovine hormone or pesticides, organic milk is almost always *ultra-pasteurized*. One of the only processes less healthy than pasteurizing your family's milk is ultra-pasteurizing that milk.

Alcohol can decrease HGH levels. Remember that alcohol is basically sugar. You've heard that some red wine can add a life-extending substance called *resveratrol* to your system. Certainly alcohol in moderation isn't going to harm you. But keep in mind that alcohol is sugar and sugar is basically toxic to your system which is why you might get drunk on a little bit of whiskey but not on the same amount of water or iced tea.

Perhaps you're tired of sugar being to blame for so many problems in this book. We are too! We wish that a 2 liter cola and a Snickers bar were healthy foods!

Actually, we've been eating so well for so long that just thinking about both of those make us sort of queasy to our stomachs. That's the good news about eating properly. Your body automatically turns on rejection mechanisms to keep you away from the bad stuff. It takes months of eating badly to wear down your rejection mechanisms and to make your hormone response so sluggish that you no longer reject those phony food items and begin to crave them. A broken body and a broken hormone balance craves sugar because the hormones are not able to sync up well enough to give you a genuine feel-good feeling so you seek outside sources than only make the problems worse.

But if for no other reason, you must get off the sugar bandwagon to look better. Yes, a piece of frozen pie from your grocer's freezer is not going to cause you long-term problems by itself. But while that pie is in your system your body will tell itself, "I should store some of this sugar because I don't need it all right now. Hmm, where would be a good place? Oh, there is room for even more fat cells on those hips, we'll stick it there."

Putting Your HGH in Balance

The formula that begins putting your HGH in balance *and keeping it there* is extremely similar to other hormones. That's the whole beauty of approaching your hormone balancing act yourself, at least before you seek medical help other than to get initial testing to see if any of your hormones are out of whack. That beauty is that hormones seem to respond negatively to many of the same things and hormone balance seems to prefer many of the same things across the whole spectrum of hormones.

You know the dietary route well by now. It's just what you expect because your body is not crazy. What is good for your body in one place is almost always good for the rest of your body.

Lots of healthy fats, good protein sources, and fibrous vegetables are the dietary key to producing a healthy dose of HGH. To the extent that you deviate and eat more sugar and less protein, or to the extent that you eat corn-based protein found in almost every USDA "meat" sold at almost every fast-food restaurant, your HGH and can be adversely affected. Protein seems to be more important even than fat for good HGH secretion so don't let your protein intake drop. Eat good protein at every meal.

Note: The fast food chain named *Chipotle* is known for its hormone-free ingredients and its grass-fed beef, pork, and cage-free chickens. Chipotle attempts to source some of its food locally throughout the United States close to the restaurant locations that use the food. They are not 100% grass-fed and cage-free but they are working towards that goal and should be commended. The movie *Food, Inc.*, is an excellent documentary showing you the poor health of the nation's FDA- and USDA-approved food supply. One of the extra features on the disc is a segment about Chipotle's food sourcing that is eye-opening. It'll make you want to load up your family tonight and take them there! Not only will your family like the taste, so will your hormones! (Go easy on the white rice.)

Routine exercise also improves your HGH production. You don't have to become a fitness guru; actually, doing too much seems to cause your hormones to react badly. But move around, go outdoors on breaks and get some sun, swim, play recreational sports with your family, and just have a moderately active lifestyle to stave off many aches, pains, and hormonal maladies that can arise faster from a sedimentary lifestyle.

Since you're going to eat better and move around more, your HGH will be happier and more productive. In addition, other hormone levels will spike to good levels and you'll sleep better too. It turns out that good sleep habits also improve HGH levels.

It's like your body's internal parts are designed to work together in a system!

Supplementing with HGH

Lots of problems arise with HGH drug supplementation.

Athletes who have abuse growth hormones can develop *acromegaly* which can result in tumors around the pituitary gland, body odor, fatigue, excess sweating, headaches, excess hair growth in women, and more.

In general, there is a good reason why even medical doctors refuse to give HGH to otherwise healthy patients who request it.

CHAPTER 10

THE SLEEP HORMONE

–

MELATONIN

Next to insulin, melatonin is one of the most widely-known hormones.

International travelers take melatonin while crossing multiple time zones in an attempt to get their sleep pattern modified for the upcoming night. Insomnia sufferers have melatonin supplements in their bathroom cabinets.

Unlike many other hormones such as HGH, melatonin supplements are available over-the-counter and when used at their intended doses provide virtually no side effects. If nothing else, hopefully the prevalence of melatonin has reduced the usage of Ambien with its reported psychedelic side-effects that lead to additional problems.

Having said that, people do pop melatonin without much thought to its intended use and it's best to approach anything like that with some knowledge.

So here is some knowledge.

How Melatonin Cycles You Up and Down

Throughout the day, your levels of melatonin secretion rise and fall. The reason is that melatonin levels change is that our activity levels change. In the optimum state, melatonin levels increase at night when we sleep and decrease during the day to keep us active. If our schedules change, such as we begin working the night-shift or switch time zones due to travel, out cycles can get out of alignment for a while until our bodies realize that they need to modify the release cycle of melatonin.

Melatonin is an antioxidant to help ward off dangerous oxidizing agents in bodies and food. As with metal that gets rusty after it comes out of water and hits oxygen, oxygen can damage your body through a normal process that a healthy diet and good levels or hormones such as melatonin inhibit. "Free radicals" form from oxidation, which attack our systems if not kept under routine check by the rest of our body.

As you age, you normally sleep less because melatonin production is reduced through the normal process of aging. Teenagers who insist on staying up late and sleeping late aren't *fully* to blame for their insistence on such a schedule because in the teen years melatonin production appears a little later at night and produces longer into the early morning hours than at other times in our lives.

There is evidence that melatonin helps protect against immunity disorders although the research is still being finalized and verified across the world.

Problems with Melatonin Imbalance

Besides a bad night's sleep, too little melatonin can result in an under-production of a hormone called cortisol, which you'll learn about in the next chapter. (Cortisol and melatonin, when not in balance, are somewhat enemies and can work against each other.)

Having to sleep in the daytime hours or having to stay awake at night after dark is more difficult due to the fact that light and darkness trigger melatonin decreases and increases. We truly are made to sleep at night when it's dark and be awake in the day when it's light.

Low melatonin has been linked to autism and premature aging. Although a lack of melatonin has not been said to be a cause, melatonin supplementation is sometimes helpful for those who suffer from migraines and cluster headaches.

Too much melatonin is rare and even when supplementation is too much the side effects have not been recorded as major at this time.

Putting Your Melatonin in Balance

Often what fixes a good night's sleep helps your melatonin production. When you sleep, even if work forces you to be a day sleeper, you want the room as dark as possible to get your body secreting melatonin. Even digital clocks and the television in an otherwise dark room can impair your melatonin production.

As stated earlier in this book, a good night's sleep not only makes you healthier, wealthier, and wise (actually, it may have been Ben Franklin who said that...), a good night's sleep has also been found to aid in weight loss. You know you feel better when you've slept well and you think better and feel better on the whole.

If you need additional help to sleep better, using a 3mg melatonin supplement such as the one found here helps for short-term sleeping problems and time-zone adjustments: http://www.amazon.com/Foods-Melatonin-High-Grade-Capsules/dp/B0019LTGC2/ref=sr_1_6?ie=UTF8&qid=1337 641689&sr=8-6.

Depending on your weight and muscle mass, up to 9mg might be necessary to achieve optimal sleep. You may have to play around with the dosage a while to see what works well for you. Don't immediately jump to 9mg if you haven't tried melatonin before, however, because taking more when you don't need it can actually inhibit your sleep cycle. My co-author, Rich, sleeps far better with 9mg but when I (Jennifer) take 9mg, at about 2AM every time the eyes open and it's a good 3 hours of being wide-awake before sleep comes once again.

Some people see better results with liquid drops instead of the tablets. You can get 2.5mg drops here: http://www.amazon.com/Natrol-Melatonin-2-5-Liquid-8-Ounce/dp/B001HCOFMO/ref=sr_1_1?s=hpc&ie=UTF8&qi d=1337937034&sr=1-1

Note: When using drops, it's suggested that you put the drop or drops under your tongue for a few seconds instead of swallowing it directly. This can raise the effectiveness of the drops by getting the melatonin into your blood supply more quickly than swallowing the melatonin.

You don't want to stay on melatonin longer than three months if it's not necessary. Actually, you don't want to stay on it for any time longer than necessary. Often, if you go a night or two with a restless night's sleep, melatonin for the next couple of nights can put your right back into your normal sleep patterns. The effects from taking melatonin for more than three months have been studied and have proven to be inconclusive. Some people have taken melatonin supplements for years and report no side effects and great sleep patterns.

So it's an individual kind of thing that you will have to gauge for yourself. But if your body can make enough melatonin, needing only a kick-start every once in a while through a supplement, then it's probably best to allow your body to do its job and leave the supplements for the exceptional occasions and long trips.

CHAPTER 11

THE STRESS HORMONE

–

CORTISOL

Your adrenal glands produce the hormone called cortisol. With adrenal problems you're often tired and down during the day and you cannot sleep at night. An adrenal hormone deficiency can give you strong cravings for chocolate. This is because your body's serotonin (the feel-good chemical in your brain) is created by the adrenal glands. Chocolate stimulates serotonin. People who crave chocolate are actually craving serotonin.

When you have anxiety, fear, or other forms of stress your body secretes more cortisol. Cortisol enables you to better handle stress. But cortisol also works with your metabolism-related system. Cortisol raises your blood sugar level when it gets too low. Your energy level is directly affected by how well balanced your cortisol level is.

Problems with Cortisol Imbalance

As you'll see in Chapter 13, a prolonged cortisol rise can work against other hormones, especially DHEA, that help offset the effects of too much cortisol. Cortisol can begin to cause damage when left unchecked.

If your body produces too much cortisol, for example, then your melatonin is reduced. The excess cortisol doesn't allow your melatonin secretions to occur naturally. Your sleep therefore becomes more difficult. Other problems soon can follow such as extended insomnia and depression.

The "happy" brain chemical called *serotonin* shuts down with too much cortisol production. Your mood will be depressed and your interest in life's normal activities can drop. Sexual problems can arise, especially lack of desire. The combination of little sleep and slower response, results in weight gain, especially around your stomach.

A lack of cortisol production, which is less common than excess cortisol, results in diarrhea which works with other factors to cause unnatural and rapid weight loss.

Out-of-balance cortisol levels can result in major diseases such as Cushing's Disease and diabetes. Cosmetically, dark circles under your eyes can appear demonstrating high cortisol levels. (Such dark circles might also be a result of HGH deficiency too.)

If you have weight gain and cannot seem to lose fat, or you have a lack of interest in daily activities and have little interest in sex, get your cortisol levels checked.

Note: Studies have shown that females are generally more attracted to males who have healthy, normally low cortisol levels over those who have elevated cortisol levels. The reason might be that low cortisol is an indicator that those men are less anxious and therefore more confident. Just thought I'd throw that in there.

Putting Your Cortisol in Balance

Sugar is a danger for cortisol-imbalanced patients. You need to avoid sugar in all forms including alcohol to try to get your cortisol levels back into their normal range. High cortisol levels are more common in people who eat fast foods and processed and pre-packaged foods because excess salt can also damage cortisol levels.

If you're eating correctly and eating a hormone-healthy lifestyle you almost certainly don't get too much salt and that sodium shouldn't be a problem even if you add it to some of your meals once in a while.

Exercise alone doesn't necessarily improve cortisol but exercise does help you deal with stress in almost all situations better, so exercise can reduce stress in your body and mind and keep cortisol functioning more normally.

Whatever you do, maintain a healthy diet full of good fats. Low-fat diets can negatively affect your cortisol levels so stay away from them at all costs the rest of your life.

Eat regularly and don't skip meals. Doing so can cause your body to literally cannibalize itself by taking muscle tissue from your leg area to be converted to glucose-based sugar fuel for energy. (Perhaps the only good news is that sometimes tissue from your butt is used instead of leg muscles (good news if you want a smaller butt!)

Note: Remember you're to eat a variety of colorful vegetables? Beets provide a dark, burgundy colored vegetable and just a half of a beet daily can clear out your stress hormones such as excess cortisol, and adrenaline. In addition, beets can help reverse our environment's heavy estrogen-inducing atmosphere full of pesticides and food made with soy. Grate one-half of a raw beet and put on a daily salad to maximize this amazing vegetable. All this from half a beet! Want a final reason to grab organic beets the next time you go shopping? They can improve your lean muscle mass, which speeds up your metabolism naturally, which makes weight loss easier.

Your Liver

Given that cortisol is a primary stress hormone, your liver can come under extreme stress when your hormones go out of balance. You can get a potbelly look in your stomach's region when your liver is out of shape. Your body looks and even feels like a water balloon because fluid is leaking… because the liver can't produce proteins. You must take your stress of liver.

One of the best methods to rejuvenate your liver can be found in *1-Day Diet: The Fastest "Diet" in the World.*

CHAPTER 12

THE HUNGER-STIMULATING HORMONE

–

GHRELIN

Your stomach and pancreas secret ghrelin... a hormone that stimulates your appetite.

In a way, ghrelin prepares you for meals because before you eat, your ghrelin increases and when you finish – if properly secreted – your ghrelin levels decrease. If you go too long without eating, your ghrelin level will rise accordingly in an effort to get you to look for food.

Actually, when you just *think* of food your ghrelin will increase in an effort to prepare you for a potential meal.

Unlike leptin which rises to make you feel satisfied after eating, a rising level of ghrelin makes you feel hungry.

When you're hungry, you typically are not depressed. Hunger is a motivator to find food and not a depressant. Therefore, indirectly ghrelin acts as a natural anti-depressant.

Problems with Ghrelin Imbalance

One reason why lack of sleep can increase your weight gain is because serotonin is a brain chemical that naturally flattens your production of ghrelin when ghrelin is unneeded. (You owe it to yourself to learn more about the important brain chemical nutrient serotonin. You can learn all about it and the other vital brain chemicals in *Brain Controlled Weight Loss*.) Without the controlling serotonin, your ghrelin stays high and you stay hungry. Fortunately, Chapter 4's hormone-healthy diet also is brain healthy and can help maintain a proper level of serotonin too.

So, when you can increase your level of serotonin you get more sleep. More sleep causes your ghrelin levels to rise. The elevated ghrelin levels do two things:

1. Boosts your HGH

2. Reduces your cravings for carbohydrates, enabling you to eat better food with higher good fats and proteins.

To help clarify what high ghrelin can do, ScienceDaily.com, one of the most popular science news websites, described an in-depth study of sleep and ghrelin funded by the National Institute of Health. ScienceDaily.com said the following in their October 4, 2010 edition:

> *Higher ghrelin levels have been shown to "reduce energy expenditure, stimulate hunger and food intake, promote retention of fat, and increase hepatic glucose production to support the availability of fuel to glucose dependent tissues," the authors note. "In our experiment, sleep restriction was accompanied by a similar pattern of increased hunger and ... reduced oxidation of fat."*

Putting Your Ghrelin in Balance

Get a restful night's sleep by supplementing with melatonin if you need to. This boosts your serotonin and keeps your ghrelin in check so that your ghrelin appears when you need to eat but then goes away. Like nosy neighbors, the hormone ghrelin is something you don't want to stick around too long after a meal.

Obviously a hormone-healthy lifestyle of eating a high-fat, high-protein, and fibrous carbohydrate diet will help ghrelin and the hormones connected with ghrelin. Everything in your body seeks to be in balance because all the parts work together to keep you alive. It's in your best interest to help your hormones. Plus you'll feel so much better and lose weight.

Note: A new vaccine is being tested that is called the *anti-obesity vaccine*. We're not too fond of this "solution" to weight loss but it's interesting to look at while discussing ghrelin. This vaccine uses your own body's immune system to suppress the production of ghrelin. This suppresses your appetite. Now with vaccines come costs: they are a non-food answer, and known sometimes to add toxic mercury to your system and such an anti-obesity vaccine working to suppress a normal and needed hormone seems like something to be avoided. Only time will tell whether or not the anti-obesity vaccine lives up to its name or not. Extremely obese patients may very well need extra help to lose initial weight. The problem comes if the obesity problem is helped and the patient loses weight, the lifestyle that enabled the obesity is going to still be present. Using a natural remedy to reduce obesity enables you to keep slim and feeling good and balanced from the start.

Again, ScienceDaily.com summed it up well when they announced:

> *"For the first time, we have evidence that the amount of sleep makes a big difference on the results of dietary interventions. One should not ignore the way they sleep when going on a diet. Obtaining adequate sleep may enhance the beneficial effects of a diet. Not getting enough sleep could defeat the desired effects."*

Two years later in 2012, ScienceDaily.com followed up with a related story entitled, *Lack of Sleep Makes Your Brain Hungry* in which they said this:

> *New research from Uppsala University shows that a specific brain region that contributes to a person's appetite sensation is more activated in response to food images after one night of sleep loss than after one night of normal sleep. Poor sleep habits can therefore affect people's risk of becoming overweight in the long run. [...]*

> *In a new study, Christian Benedict, together with Samantha Brooks, Helgi Schiöth and Elna-Marie Larsson from Uppsala University and researchers from other European universities, have now systematically examined which regions in the brain, involved in appetite sensation, are influenced by acute sleep loss. By means of magnetic imaging (fMRI) the researchers studied the brains of 12 normal-weight males while they viewed images of foods. The researchers compared the results after a night with normal sleep with those obtained after one night without sleep. [...]*

> *"After a night of total sleep loss, these males showed a high level of activation in an area of the brain that is involved in a desire to eat. Bearing in mind that insufficient sleep is a growing problem in modern society, our results may explain why poor sleep habits can affect*

people's risk to gain weight in the long run. It may therefore be important to sleep about eight hours every night to maintain a stable and healthy body weight."

CHAPTER 13

THE REBUILDING HORMONE

–

DHEA

DHEA is an abbreviation for the hormone called *dehydroepiandrosterone*. Your adrenal gland produces DHEA. Like cortisol, DHEA is a stress hormone although DHEA and cortisol often find themselves working against each other as the way they handle stress differs.

DHEA could be considered a rebuilding hormone that begins to go to work when stress hits whereas cortisol does more damage when stress is present. This doesn't mean that cortisol is bad to have. The "damage" is a healthy damage that helps you eliminate some cell waste but too much cortisol certainly can be bad as you saw in Chapter 11.

Combined with too little DHEA to help offset the damage your body can get into trouble.

As always you want all your hormones to work in harmony by being at their optimum balance levels.

Problems with DHEA Imbalance

Stress, anxiety, fear, and worry all contribute to DHEA (as well as cortisol and other hormone) imbalances. With normal levels of stress, offset by a good diet and moderate exercise, your DHEA levels to rise and then fall back when the stress dampens. Too much stress causes your body to increase production of cortisol at the expense of DHEA... producing too little of the rebuilding DHEA and too much of the tearing-down cortisol. The big problem is that your body might become incapable of reducing the cortisol levels or increasing your DHEA once the stress finally goes away.

> **Note:** Another problem is that we tend to think of only one kind of stress. That is the stress that comes from life such as working too hard, worry, and so on. But physical accidents, surgery, and blood sugar changes cause your body to go through stress too. Your body responds the same way no matter what the stress source happens to be: DHEA and cortisol increases for a while to try to deal with the stress together but your DHEA gives up quickly and begins to drop to dangerously low levels while that cortisol just keeps on damaging.

You might have heard that prolonged stress makes you susceptible to disease and a DHEA imbalance is one of the key reasons why. Lowered DHEA (again, commonly accompanied with higher cortisol levels that don't drop properly) will put you at risk for all of the following problems:

- Immune system weakness

- Rising blood sugar levels

- Sodium and water retention

- High blood pressure

- Increased heart disease risk due to higher triglycerides

- Broken thyroid gland operation

- Increased belly fat

- Protein breakdown problems resulting in bone density problems

- There are more but need we go on? You want your DHEA in balance.

Too much DHEA over an extended period of time is rare except for people who over-supplement with DHEA. Acne is the primary side-effect to watch for.

Putting Your DHEA in Balance

Guess what can cause a dangerous reduction in DHEA? Eating too many grains and having too much sugar. Guess what most people eat too much of?

If you've been a cereal and bread kind of person for as long as you can remember, and a salivary DHEA-cortisol test shows low levels of DHEA, before you worry about other corrective actions stop the grains *now*. Give yourself a month off grains and retest to see if there is any movement in your DHEA.

Allergies to various grains such as wheat and rye are far more prevalent than we used to think. Four decades of the government's FDA telling you to eat more grains than anything else will catch up to all of us eventually. It has caught up. The number of gluten and grain allergies is becoming an epidemic.

Oh, and long-term soy reduces the DHEA level in some people. Look in your kitchen cabinet at any package or can. Look at another. See how many list "soy" in some form or another. Then toss every one of those things in the garbage and go buy real food from a local farmer or produce stand.

If your diet is good, then the chances are high that stress is the primary genesis of your low DHEA levels. Reducing your stress is the key. You do that through changing your lifestyle-related stress factors such as:

- Getting more sleep, perhaps by supplementing with melatonin

- Reducing your workload

- Getting help dealing with family matters that may be causing strife

Sometimes stress factors that impact us are not in our control. So if you cannot reduce your lifestyle stress, and even if you can, you need to build up your body's resistance to stress. The way you do that is through exercise and diet. Adding fermented foods such as homemade kefir, yogurt, and cold-processed sauerkraut also help strengthen your family's resistance.

Yes, the same diet this book has been promoting since the beginning is what you need. A hormone-healthy diet. Good fats and proteins amplify your resistance to stress by enabling your body to respond strongly against stress. When flare-ups occur, a body that is more immune to that stress will deal with the stress, amplifying DHEA and cortisol together properly to help you reduce the stress's physical impact on you, and once reduced those levels will return to normal.

Note: If you find, through a doctor's or nutritionist's test, that your DHEA is reduced there are several factors that your doctor should check for. Arthritis can produce low DHEA levels as can other common inflammatory problems that occur throughout people's lives. If inflammation or arthritis is ruled out, you may have a bacterial infection in your stomach. In that case you need antibiotics and you don't see us recommending antibiotics willy-nilly. Certainly, on this one listen to your doctor because drugs can effectively correct stomach bacterial infections and you don't want them to manifest into more severe problems.

CHAPTER 14

A QUICK INTRODUCTION TO YOUR SEX-RELATED HORMONES

One of the most important aspects of hormonal balance comes to light when it comes to sexual functioning.

Hormones are *everything* when it comes to sex drive with the rare exceptions of a physical (structural) problem or something internal such as endometriosis flaring up and making sex painful and unwanted. Of course emotional and relationship problems are often the cause of so many sexual problems but surprisingly some of those can melt once one fixes internal hormonal problems such as estrogen or testosterone deficiencies or abundances.

The next three chapters focus primarily on these hormones:

- Estrogen

- Progesterone

- Testosterone

Even if You Don't Miss the Sex

If you have no sex drive but you are happy with that and so is your spouse, or if you live alone and don't want a sex drive, you should understand that a healthy sex drive *is a sign of a healthy body* and the opposite is true also. No sex drive is often a major indicator of health problems. These problems often manifest themselves in sexual problems early before building to even more serious conditions later.

In most books covering hormones, the sexual hormones cover some of the greatest amount of real estate because of their leading indication status for other problems. This book is going to be an exception to that, however. We're going to focus on a general state of healthiness and sexual function that typically accompany normal levels of the sexual hormones.

We're going to discuss what happens if you're too low or too high on those hormones and look for ways to balance them again. We're not going into all the ins and outs and possibilities simply because this is a vast region and for typical health and weight loss you just don't need the scientific depth that you can find elsewhere if you want that.

Sexual Supplements

Certainly supplements can play a major role in balancing the sex hormones. Unlike HGH and some others, sexual hormone supplementation through prescriptions have been quite effective. (Some have been quite horrid too.) We won't ignore the supplementation issues but given the focus of health and weight loss we will refer you to other sources for more in-depth and serious coverage of those issues.

So for the next two chapters we'll focus on the balance of your sexual hormones and some of the more common and healthy ways to try to put them into balance through routine, healthy, natural methods.

CHAPTER 15

THE SEX HORMONES FOR WOMEN

In general, and this is only a rule of thumb, if you and your spouse love each other but have *any* problems sexually where disinterest of one party or the other is involved, then there is a brain nutrient or hormone problem. Yes, it can be emotional but hormones often trigger emotions that get blamed for such problems. Yes, it can be physical and it can be emotional and it's always wise to get everything checked. But assume that physical issues are not the primary culprit until a professional determines otherwise.

For our purposes, a lack of desire and even physical pain of sex (such as endometriosis) can very well have origins in hormonal imbalances.

Hormones determine your sex drive above all other factors.

Obviously estrogen is a primary female sex hormone that needs to be discussed but healthy women also have low levels of testosterone (low relative to healthy men) and progesterone levels are also extremely critical. All three hormones need to be in balance for you, if female, to desire a healthy amount of sex. And a desire for sex is a primary sign of health so it's one that needs to be analyzed by a professional in almost every case. We'll work on fixing your hormones primarily by diet here but you should also seek help from a nutritionist-aware physician.

Menopause is Often a Problem Solved Badly

So many factors exist to consider that we have to narrow them down here to stay focused on your weight and general well-being. One of the most obvious evidences of a hormonal problem in women as they hit middle age is menopause. Menopausal women often find that their weight gain skyrockets and just gets out of control, perhaps for the first time in their lives.

If nothing has changed other than you've gotten older and your weight is up, you must remember that hormones affect your biochemistry directly. And the word *biochemistry* begins with *bio* and *bios* in Greek means *life*. The center of life's universe on earth is sex. That is where life begins and so that should be a primary focus of health. Don't shrug off menopausal weight gain or a growing lack of interest in sex as normal aging. Your very quality of *life* is on the line.

> **Note:** Yes, as we age it *is* normal that we find it harder to lose weight than when we were young and were extremely active and when our muscles were larger from work and exercise which burned calories more favorably than our lessened muscle mass in middle age and beyond. Yes, as we age it *is* normal to see a decrease in our sex drives. But if either reaches even a minor "problem" stage, and let's face it we *do* often intuitively know when that is, we must suspect hormones and also get checked by someone who understands hormones and health.

Many people, especially women, attack their aging weight problem with calorie-restrictive diets. As we've discussed before in this book (and especially in our *Brain Controlled Weight Loss* volume), restricting your calories does the following:

1. Makes you lose water weight quickly. (Almost *any* "diet" when followed will do this initially. That is why it's such as red herring making people believe they are following a good diet when it may be extremely dangerous as many calorie-restrictive diets are.)

2. Puts your body into long-term starvation mode which puts your hormones in a tizzy like they've never seen before. This causes energy to be taken away from vital organs such as your liver in an attempt to keep you alive just a little longer after the lack of food for fuel.

3. Once you fall off the calorie-restriction diet, and you will, you gain the weight back and more due to your body's extreme craving at that moment for instant fuel that comes from horrible carbohydrates such as mashed potatoes, chips, bread, sweets, and other "comfort" foods that don't comfort your body but that do spike your body's blood sugar level.

Menopause itself comes about because of hormonal changes. You cannot stop it from happening of course, and you wouldn't want to if someone finds a way. Menopause is a normal function in a healthy life. But you can minimize the negatives and maximize your health in all other ways, including your weight, by understanding which hormones are most susceptible and ways to work on normalizing them as much as possible.

Problems with Female Sex Hormone Imbalances

Aging affects the presence of a balance of female-related hormones such as estrogen and progesterone. If only aging was the only problem to deal with. Contraception can possibly disrupt your hormones which is why you want to be checked carefully throughout your use of them. Caffeine affects your sex hormonal balance as can alcohols and other sugars and starchy and sugary carbohydrates. Not surprisingly to these authors, fat-free dairy has been shown to be a major disruptor of female hormones.

> **Note:** No, since you began reading this book the government *still* has not changed its stance on promoting a low-fat diet.

So many things in the environment mimic hormones and estrogen mimicking is one of the worst culprits both for men and women.

Pesticides, soy, and preservatives in thousands of food products mimic the injection of our systems with substances that our bodies react to the same way they would react to excess estrogen production in our own glands.

> **Note:** The World Health Organization, a governing body that seemingly wants more and more power if you look at its policies and recommendations, says that these parabens (estrogen look-a-likes) are low risk factors and can be ignored. The reason they state this is that parabens are up to 100,000 less potent than estrogen-related hormones so they pose little danger. That may very well be but what they fail to note is that these parabens appear in quantities up to *one million times the quantity of the estrogen-related hormones!* (This

comes from the Journal of Applied Toxicology, March, 2012.) Therefore, by the WHO's own published standards, these estrogen-mimicking parabens are present at levels *ten times higher* than normal estrogen-like hormones factors. This poses a real danger to women. High estrogen levels are not always, and perhaps rarely, a result of the human body's own functioning. You need to be constantly aware of this as you buy your food. The next time you pass up organic produce over conventional, consider the risks. These parabens also appear in heavy quantities in deodorants and guess what? Breast cancer often begins in the underarm areas! So you owe it to yourself to seek a natural deodorant for you and your family.

Increased estrogen exposure is most dangerous to children. Children as young as eight years old are experiencing puberty in record numbers over the past 2 decades. Why is that? Certainly it's not evolution. It has to be environmental.

By the way, *ginger* has properties shown to reduce this paraben toxicity according to a paper recently published by R.J. Verma from the University School of Sciences in Gujart University, India. As an added bonus, and a big bonus at that, ginger has incredible properties to maximize your brain's functioning as we describe in *Brain Controlled Weight Loss – The Solution to Failed Diets & Exercise Programs.*

For women, an imbalance of estrogen can portend serious issues such as:

- Weight gain (of course)

- Sexual dysfunction and desire issues

- Migraine headaches

- Tenderness in the breasts

- Infertility issues

- Uterine cancer

- Endometriosis

- Strokes

- Heart problems

- Decreased vaginal lubrication

And this list is far from exhaustive.

The hormone progesterone is also a problem when it's out of balance even though it doesn't get the press that estrogen does. Progesterone helps regulate menstrual cycles, pregnancy, and embryo formation. In addition, progesterone works to help regulate estrogen. Again, here is an example of one hormone that needs to be in balance to help keep another hormone in balance. You cannot focus on single hormones in your body which is why we have tried to address the entire group through diet primarily first throughout this book.

Progesterone imbalances can occur and when they do you may see signs of:

- Weight gain (of course); an over-abundance of estrogen can shift fat from your butt to your belly.

- Depression

- Period disruptions

- Menstrual problems such as excess bleeding

- Cysts in the breasts

- Too large of a chest (that's possible even for women!) may be an indicator of progesterone problems.

A Professional Weighs In

Recently, Dr. Joseph Mercola, MD, told his subscribers of the horrid impact of parabens and concluded with this which we can find absolutely nothing to argue with:

- ***Radically reduce your sugar/fructose intake.***
  Normalizing your insulin levels by avoiding sugar and fructose is one of the most powerful physical actions you can take to lower your risk of cancer. Unfortunately, very few oncologists appreciate or apply this knowledge today. The Cancer Centers of America is one of the few exceptions, where strict dietary measures are included in their cancer treatment program. Fructose is especially dangerous, as research shows it actually speeds up cancer growth.

- ***Optimize your vitamin D level.*** *Ideally it should be over 50 ng/ml, but levels from 70-100 ng/ml will radically reduce your cancer risk. Safe sun exposure is the most effective way to increase your levels, followed by safe tanning beds and then oral vitamin D3 supplementation as a last resort if no other option is available.*

- ***Maintain a healthy body weight.*** *This will come naturally when you begin eating right for your nutritional type* *and exercising using high-intensity burst-type activities[...]. It's important to lose excess weight because estrogen is produced in fat tissue.*

- **Get plenty of high quality animal-based omega-3 fats,** *such as those from krill oil. Omega-3 deficiency is a common underlying factor for cancer.*

- **Avoid drinking alcohol,** *or limit your drinks to one a day for women.*

- **Breastfeed exclusively for up to six months.** *Research shows this will reduce your breast cancer risk.*

- **Watch out for excessive iron levels.** *This is actually very common once women stop menstruating. The extra iron actually works as a powerful oxidant, increasing free radicals and raising your risk of cancer. So if you are a post-menopausal woman or have breast cancer you will certainly want to have your Ferritin level drawn. Ferritin is the iron transport protein and should not be above 80. If it is elevated you can simply donate your blood to reduce it.*

By the way, high iron is also a problem for men and it often goes undetected due to men's common lack of requesting regular full-spectrum blood tests. Men never menstruate and most don't get cuts and scrapes the way our forefathers who worked outdoors got. The best way for men to keep their iron levels at healthy levels also helps others: Men should give blood regularly. This is usually all that's needed to maintain a healthy level of iron.

Testosterone Isn't Just for Men

Women need testosterone to function normally just as men need some estrogen. The problem, as always, is balance.

If you have been showing signs of a low sex drive, obviously you need to begin the hormone-healthy diet lifestyle immediately but you also need to get all your sexual hormone levels checked by a professional. Medical treatment of low levels of testosterone differs from that of, say, low levels of estrogen. (Fortunately, if diet alone will put your sexual functioning hormones back in balance, the same diet works well for all three: estrogen, progesterone, and testosterone. In addition, some other factors you'll learn about below will also help adjust them into better ranges.)

If your glands are producing too much testosterone, you could experience hair loss where you don't want it and hair growth where you don't want that! (Conjure up an image of a bald guy with a beard...) In addition your voice can deepen. Worse, you'll have a tendency to put on shoulder pads, try out for the team, and pat your teammates on the backside after each touchdown.

Note: We actually have no technical, scientific, or medical evidence that any of that last part will occur.

Too little testosterone in women might at first seem to be a minor thing but the health problems related to low testosterone comprises a surprisingly complete list including:

- No sex drive and/or no orgasms

- Pain during sex

- Premature aging

- Depression and related disorders such as severe fear and depression

- Vaginal itching

- Muscle atrophy

Low-fat diets can reduce your testosterone so stay away from those.

Putting Your Female Sex Hormones in Balance

First of all, a diet high in good fats goes a long way towards staving off these hormonal problems. Keep your protein up and consider eating some oysters if you can due to their impact, although somewhat minor, on testosterone levels.

A group of vegetables from the cruciferous family acts as both an estrogen-reducing agent and an antitoxin. These vegetables are all low in carbohydrates and include:

- Cabbage

- Broccoli

- Cauliflower

- Radish

- Kale

- Brussels sprouts

You must make a major inspection of your cosmetic sources as well as your food sources to help reduce the problems society finds itself having these days. Moving to a natural deodorant is a must and if you can find one without *any* aluminum (or alum) you will also keep more of that heavy metal from your system.

If you don't overdose on it, green tea actually has some positive effects on female hormones.

Estrogen rarely is considered to be too low these days with all the hormone-mimicking estrogen, but it can occur. If you end up accepting a doctor's advice to get estrogen treatments, get a second opinion. If you then trust both opinions get bio-identical female hormone replacements. These *are* considered as safe as possible given the data we currently have. If it's not bio-identical, stay completely away as if it is pure poison.

Finally, a treatment that will make your husband jump for joy. More sex will increase your testosterone naturally. Obviously if you have pain then you might not be able to pursue this avenue until some of the other possible solutions kick in, but once you are able to you should begin trying sex once again… even if the desire isn't quite there yet. Go through the motions to help stimulate your testosterone levels and increase the speed at which your desire returns.

Note: Zinc is a good supplement for improving your sex hormone balances. Zinc plays a big role in fertility.

CHAPTER 16

THE SEX HORMONES FOR MEN

Note: For those men reading this book who jumped directly to this chapter first, we understand! Still, there is so much critical information before this that you need to know before this chapter can be effective. Chapter 4's dietary plan for healthy hormones is a must-read especially before you read this chapter.

Men, certainly the hormone testosterone is a major hormone for you and the lifestyle you want to live. Testosterone literally defines you just as estrogen defines women. The thing you may not have known before is that your body, if healthy, also produces estrogen and progesterone. Your estrogen and progesterone levels, although far less than healthy levels for females, are critical to keep in balance.

With aging brings a lowered sex drive naturally. That typically isn't a huge deal for men as long as the frequency remains in numbers that differ from man to man but as long as the desire still remains and everything functions normally. If you begin to worry that things are no longer functioning normally, or if your desire seems to be far weaker than it has been in the distant past, then hormonal changes are almost certainly to be looked at.

Through a simple blood test doctors can check for your testosterone, estrogen, and progesterone levels. The results will let you know if one or more of those hormones are too weak or too strong.

It's true that the Erectile Dysfunction drugs have made a major impact on society today. It's also true that ED may very well be only a symptom and not a cause. Treating ED when a symptom and not the cause can rob you of a far more healthy *and active* life in all ways including sexually. The cause can often be, you guessed it, hormonal.

Problems with Male Sex Hormone Imbalances

Looking at testosterone first, abnormally low levels obviously can produce sexual dysfunction. Other than a gradual reduction due to aging, a more rapid decrease might signal a drop in testosterone production. You need to immediately fix your lifestyle to help the levels boost back up. (In severe drops you may very well need hormone replacement therapy, see below. Surprisingly, other than being somewhat costly without insurance, this treatment is fairly benign and has proved to work well in men.)

Not only will you have a lowered sex drive with lowered testosterone, you'll have the tendency to put on weight, especially around your middle stomach section. Middle age weight gain is not something you should focus on first as you now know well enough if you've read the book up to this point. You need to focus on your hormone levels first or you may never reduce that spare tire around your middle.

In addition to a low sex drive, erectile dysfunction, and weight gain, low testosterone levels can lead to:

- Looking far older than your actual age

- Indecisiveness

- Depression and related disorders such as anxiety and fear

- Decreased muscle mass which helps speed up your weight gain even further

- Wrinkles which aids in making you look even older than low testosterone already makes you look

Perhaps not surprisingly, the lack of confidence and indecisiveness may be why studies show women are more attracted to men with higher testosterone levels than low levels. Not only do pheromones probably transmit this fact to their unconscious receptors, your lack of confidence is almost always a negative for women when it comes to traits they look for in men. (See Chapter 11 for more on this phenomenon and how another hormone called cortisol also factors into this.)

If you get too much testosterone, which normally comes from athletes who overdose on it and from non-monitoring by prescribing physicians, you will experience these symptoms:

- Dramatically increased urination

- Enlarged prostate

- Baldness (baldness can occur naturally from regular healthy levels of testosterone too due to genetics; bald uncles on your mother's side of the family are especially leading indicators that you have a natural tendency to lose hair more rapidly than you otherwise might)

Estrogen and Progesterone Aren't Just for Women Anymore

It's true that you men are not 100% raging testosterone machines. You are machines that, when healthy, also produce estrogen and progesterone and you need both of those although in smaller quantities than testosterone.

When your estrogen levels are at high levels you can probably guess at the symptoms already. They are typically the opposite of a high testosterone situation and include:

- Abnormally large breasts (manboobs)

- Prostate trouble that leads to extreme urination frequencies

- Lowered sperm counts

- Higher voice

- Less facial and body hair

- Feminine characteristics in the way you project yourself

The problem with high estrogen levels is not usually that you produce too much. The problem is that it's the paraben-laced environment and your diet that can be, and often is, responsible for the feminization of men today from high estrogen levels. Through pesticides and an abundance of soy in almost every processed food that you eat, as well as an abundance of soy fed to cattle and chickens that were never designed to digest soy, you are getting tons of the stuff whether you want it or not.

Unless you want to sing soprano in the Tabernacle Choir, skip back to the previous chapter and read if it you skipped it before. Yes, it's for women but you'll see some scary information there about how men, women, and worst of all children, are getting bombarded with estrogen in levels that are ten times too high *for women*. And those levels are astronomical for men and children.

> **Note:** A blood test can tell you if you're low or high in estrogen, low that is for a male. Such a problem is extremely rare. This is perhaps due to the major environmental and dietary influences just mentioned.

Just as too little estrogen in men rarely occurs, fortunately too much progesterone occurs only in extremely rare cases. Most of the time an imbalance of progesterone in men occurs on the high side. This can affect your prostate negatively as well as give you symptoms of anxiety, excess fears, and nervousness.

Prostate Issues

It is said that:

> Men either die *of* prostate problems or *with* prostate problems.

If you think about that for a bit, it seems as though prostate problems are inevitable and it's just a matter of when and how much. Although this may be true to some extent given the natural processes that occur in men as you age, it's almost always agreed that you don't have to die of prostate cancer in most cases. The easiest way is to avoid it altogether. The easiest way to do that is through diet. (You knew we would say that, right?)

Pumpkin seeds are good for keeping your prostate happy and eating them daily is never a bad thing. Obviously, avoid the pesticides which will offset any advantages of the pumpkin seeds. Buy organic.

Supplements can help ward off prostate problems too. It's widely known that saw palmetto (and nettle root which often comes with saw palmetto supplements) can help keep a prostate well but also omega-3 oils found in big numbers in Chapter 4's dietary lifestyle also work well towards keeping your prostate in good shape. In addition, the heart-healthy CoQ10 has been shown to have good effects on the prostate.

These supplements at LifeExtension.com contain some advanced supplement formulations for those of you who want to ward off problems later not only through diet but also through supplementation: http://www.lef.org/search/health-goal.prostate/index.aspx

An advantage of LifeExtension's choice of prostate supplements, over straight saw palmetto which is usually what is used, is that they are rich in a variety of supplements that are overall good for other functions in your body too.

Putting Your Male Sex Hormones in Balance

It's easy to imagine Party Guy right? You know, he's the one who has a drink in one hand and a new girl in the other. The problem with that image, as college students sometimes find out in an embarrassing way, is that alcohol lowers your testosterone *and* raises your estrogen levels by causing a conversion of some testosterone to estrogen. Lower testosterone lowers your desirability in women as mentioned earlier. To compound this problem, alcohol also increases your stress hormone cortisol. And remember, as mentioned earlier, higher cortisol levels and lower testosterone combine to cause women to be less attracted to men. So alcohol is a double-whammy for your sexual functioning.

Since alcohol is a sugar, sugary foods can put your hormones out of balance. (So can an excess in caffeine by the way. Coffee can increase your body's conversion of testosterone to estrogen by as much as 60%.) (And don't get us *started* on putting sugar *in* coffee, we could go on for hours!)

The next time you consider a second helping of pie – or even the *first* helping! – consider what that sugar will do to your testosterone and other sexual hormones. Only then should you decide if you want that pie or not.

We're not trying to use scare tactics (not *really* trying) but sugar is a toxin and the levels we eat carbs at today is simply unacceptable. It's so easy to say, "Just one," or "I've been good for a few days so I'll eat a little." We owe it to ourselves to remember that sugar is like toxin to our systems and simple carbs such as pasta and most breads and potatoes and grains such as corn turn into sugar rapidly. They are sort-of sugars as far as our blood insulin levels go.

Yes, our bodies certainly can handle sugar once in a while without much of an effect. And if we truly save dessert and an extra piece of fruit or two and for special occasions then all is well. But we fool ourselves too often. Most of the time we really do need to say "No" to sugars and simple carbs. Your weight and more important your sex hormones will *always* be better when you say "No" and will *never* be improved when you say "Yes."

A balanced high fat, high protein, low carb lifestyle as laid out in Chapter 4 is what you can do yourself to maximize your sexual hormone balance and make you the stud you know you are. Drink whole milk, raw if possible. Eat oysters and fish whose vitamins such as E seem to improve a man's hormonal balance, plenty of good beef and chicken and eggs, and maintain a healthy level of fats from good oils, nuts, and seeds. As you add good fat especially you should notice a quick increase in your sex drive if hormonal imbalance was the problem.

> **Note:** You should also emphasize eggs. Saturated fats and cholesterol-rich foods such as eggs play important roles in the production of sex hormones, especially for men. By the way, your body produces cholesterol. Your cholesterol doesn't increase with foods high in cholesterol no matter what the government's FDA has said for decades. 50% of heart attacks happen to people with "normal" cholesterol levels. Your brain *requires* cholesterol. While cholesterol can play a negative role when it's at extremely high levels, it isn't the bad guy it's made out to be. Many cultures have much higher levels of cholesterol than Americans, for example, yet have fewer heart attacks.

When Diet Isn't Enough

If diet alone doesn't seem to be enough, get a blood test to determine your testosterone, estrogen, and progesterone levels and see if more is needed. Supplements are available to help. B-complex vitamins are super and zinc specifically targets the sex hormones and seems to improve the levels.

With zinc, take about 100mg a day as a hormone balancing supplement. Zinc inhibits the aromatase enzyme that converts testosterone to estrogen. You want that enzyme! At 100mg a day, zinc also helps block the conversion of your testosterone to DHT which is a hormone that increases your chance to begin balding.

When it comes to testosterone replacement, it's actually fairly common and easy *and seems to be fairly safe* as long as your doctor monitors your levels. If you're middle age or older and you accept a natural testosterone replacement such as *Androgel 1.62%*, there are some negative side effects but they are rare and you want to be on the constant lookout that you don't start regaining too much testosterone. Too much can result in anger issues that can skyrocket out of control before you know it at the regret of you and everybody around you later. Talk to your prescribing doctor about the problems that can occur and stay in contact every few months for a check to make sure that the levels you're prescribed are keeping you at the levels your physician approves of. Reducing or increasing the rate of application is supposed to be a minor adjustment so there's little reason not to maintain a proper level.

> **Note:** One of the side effects most commonly written about, and that was actually made popular in an episode of the medical show *House*, is that anybody on hormone treatments such as testosterone replacement needs to make sure that he is the *only one getting the treatment!* In other words, you don't want to allow any part of your body where you

apply the treatment to come in contact with other members of your family, wives *and children especially*, because testosterone can be transmitted from you to them. Generally, the patch or gel is applied to an area normally covered such as your shoulder area. Even a thin shirt is adequate. As long as you wash that area first, another family member such as your wife can put her head on your shoulder at night with no worry. But you need to know that this can be a major problem for your family if you don't monitor your place of contact.

Many of the modern testosterone replacement hormones are natural and not fully synthetic (these are not bio-identical though, like the good estrogen for women is). Still they appear to have excellent results with no statistical side effects. Monitor your blood levels closely the first few months and make sure you avoid direct skin contact with others in your family on the area where you apply the hormone.

CHAPTER 17

THE ADRENALINE HORMONE

–

EPINEPHRINE

Epinephrine, more commonly known as *adrenaline*, is produced by your adrenal gland. Obviously epinephrine is a heart-related hormone because when you get excited or afraid, your heart rate rises and that's due to your body increasing your adrenaline to help prepare you for a fight-or-flight situation.

Epinephrine also helps to regulate other fight-or-flight factors such as breathing (by actually adjusting your air passage sizing) and your metabolism. When epinephrine/adrenaline is pumping, your metabolism is in high gear too! Epinephrine also affects your liver, muscles, as well as your entire system.

Epinephrine is often used as a drug, especially under emergency conditions such as cardiac arrest. People who experience anaphylactic shock and high allergy risk patients are often given epinephrine to react to the attack and try to restore their bodies to a more normal state.

Note: Jennifer's mother is severely allergic to fresh fish. She carries an *EpiPen* (a ballpoint pen-like injection system that contains epinephrine) with her at all times in case she accidentally eats something that produces an allergic reaction. That reaction is often a severe restriction in her lungs and the "adrenaline-pumping" action of the epinephrine might very well be life-saving if this occurs.

Problems with an Epinephrine Imbalance

Obviously this book isn't concerned with the trauma-related requirements of epinephrine.

Our focus here is getting and keeping our hormones in balance. Epinephrine has an effect on weight gain so it's worth knowing something about it and its cousin norepinephrine in the next chapter.

Too much epinephrine causes you to gain weight. When your life is on the line, who cares about a massive injection of epinephrine? Otherwise you don't want to trigger an increase in epinephrine if you can help it.

Drinking too much coffee or tea is one of the most common causes of spiking epinephrine. When you drink coffee, you stimulate your body through your nervous system. Sometimes we like the added "lift" that caffeine gives us. Sometimes athletes find that their performance is maximized with a little caffeine before an event. Some of us just need a little help waking up.

Note: If you're one who needs coffee to get your motor going in the mornings, you are probably addicted to it or not getting a restful night's sleep. If you drink more than three cups daily, especially non-espresso type of coffee such as the traditional cup of coffee Americans prefer which has high caffeine, you need to cut down and you probably need to look into melatonin to make your sleep more productive. Drink coffee if you like it, that's fine. Coffee has antioxidant effects on our bodies. But moderation is the key. And always buy organic.

Diet pills are often loaded with caffeine. When you eat less, your metabolism will normally slow down because you have less fuel. Dangerous calorie-restriction diets often reduce metabolism to levels so low the dieter ends up binging severely several days because their bodies crave calories and energy so badly and has gone into a starvation mode. The diet pills with caffeine jump-starts your nervous system which forces your adrenals to raise your epinephrine levels.

Although this process increases your metabolism for a short while, it does so chemically through the elevated epinephrine and not through real fuel such as real food. Insulin production increases and your blood sugar levels increase enough to give you some energy but you'll quickly die back down when the epinephrine stops pumping. This letdown feeling will make you search for more and more coffee, and eventually you'll need energy *fast* such as a candy bar or (worse because people think it's good for them) a granola bar.

Your weight and your hormone imbalance won't be helped when that continued exit of epinephrine forces you to seek sugary carbs.

Note: Anybody who has found themselves in the middle of a crime felt their adrenaline skyrocket. Afterwards they often find that they feel wobbly and weaker than they've ever felt. The dramatic epinephrine reduction after the event drains them to new low levels.

Putting Your Epinephrine in Balance

For one thing, stay away from the diet pills to adjust your epinephrine!

Also, watch your caffeine intake. A little caffeine is fine. A lot of caffeine is not good.

Also, stay away from active crime scenes!

Seriously, the best way to avoid over-stimulating your own body with epinephrine is to keep your caffeine levels under control. Three cups of coffee is the outside maximum you should drink on a regular basis. Again, the espresso and cappuccino coffees have less caffeine than American coffee and you might get away with a little more of those if you really love the stuff (as one of the authors does!).

> **Note:** Normally, pesticides are used at extreme levels when growing coffee beans. You are stacking up your hormonal disadvantages if you don't drink organic coffee. Another disadvantage of too much coffee, by the way, is increased cortisol secretion. Whoever thought to sell caffeine as a primary component of "diet pills" sure found a way to fool the public!

Don't *you* be fooled into thinking that caffeine is a dieter's dream-come-true.

But don't blame just the coffee. Again, in small amounts it would be unfair to disparage this favored drink.

Caffeine comes in many forms and drinks. Although green tea is lower in caffeine than black tea typically, and although green tea has some bonus antioxidant health benefits, you also don't want to overdose on tea throughout the day. In addition, colas are loaded with caffeine, yet another reason to consider them as helpful to your body as drinking battery acid. And just because soda is clear doesn't mean it is caffeine free. Mountain Dew has an ample supply of caffeine.

CHAPTER 18

ANOTHER FIGHT-OR-FLIGHT HORMONE

–

NOREPINEPHRINE

Norepinephrine is a cousin to epinephrine.

Norepinephrine is also known as just *norepi, NE,* and *noradrenaline.* When your norepinephrine is elevated your heart's contractions increase.

Norepinephrine usually appears in conjunction with epinephrine (adrenaline) in reaction to a fight-or-flight situation. The norepinephrine focuses on your heart the most, adjusting the heart's pumping action as needed. In addition to that, norepinephrine increases the blood to your muscles to prepare for whatever happens next as well as releases glucose from your cells for instant fuel.

All of this happens almost instantly in a healthy body when danger or extreme excitement arises (such as winning the lottery). (If you are ever told you've just won millions in the lottery, we have a piece of advice: resist the urge to fight *or* fly until you've signed the receipt for your money!)

Problems with a Norepinephrine Imbalance

The problems of too much norepinephrine mirror those of too much epinephrine discussed in the previous chapter. Again, caffeine is a common culprit that is a traditional stimulate for excess norepinephrine release which results in weight gain ultimately.

An upset in someone's production of norepinephrine in extreme cases can result in brain disorders including schizophrenia, depression, and severe ADD.

Putting Your Norepinephrine in Balance

Yep, everything in the previous chapter on epinephrine holds true for norepinephrine.

Reduce your caffeine if you're ingesting too much.

There are ways to improve your norepinephrine balance. If you've been diagnosed with one of the more serious brain problems mentioned in the previous section, you probably already are on antidepressants. We're no fan of those but we do realize there are extreme cases that need them. Antidepressants can restore levels of norepinephrine which is a primary reason they sometimes show results.

In general, you probably don't need to get tested for a norepinephrine imbalance barring some problem like a brain-related disease.

Instead, just do what you need to do daily to keep your norepinephrine and all your other hormones in good order. It shouldn't surprise you that the following foods are helpful for norepinephrine in particular:

- Eggs

- Meat

- Nuts

Isn't that interesting?

The very diet discussed in this whole book, a good fat and good animal protein-based diet is good for norepinephrine just as it is the other hormones in your system.

Vitamin B6 can also help put norepinephrine and epinephrine back to good levels but you'll find B6 in beans, meat, chicken, and fish so there's little reason to supplement if you eat well.

CHAPTER 19

THE ADDITIONAL GROWTH HORMONE

–

IGF-1

The *insulin-like growth factor* hormone is often abbreviated *IGF-1*. It's also called *somatomedin C*. Your pituitary gland secrets IGF-1. From the name *insulin-like* growth hormone, you shouldn't be surprised to learn that IGF-1 is similar in structure to insulin.

IGF-1 called is secreted during our growing years so children can grow.

You want IGF-1 to be healthy if you're overweight because IGF-1 is a fat-burning hormone (along with HGH, glucagon, epinephrine, the thyroids T3 and T4, and testosterone).

Problems with an IGF-1 Imbalance

IGF-1 production naturally decreases as we age. We don't need the growth spurts we get in childhood and our activity levels naturally decrease as we age so our bodies don't produce as much IGF-1 because our bodies simply don't need the levels they once had. In spite of it being natural, the drawback of the slowing down of IGF-1 is that it ages us. Our cells break down and die, resulting in aging of our bodies.

If your pituitary gland begins to produce too little IGF-1, all of the following can begin to occur:

- You gain weight

- Your brain gets less blood impairing your critical thinking skills and causing you to react more slowly to stimuli; in addition to slowing your brain down your memory begins to fail and your IQ begins to suffer

- Depression appears as well as related problems such as anxiety, fear, and severe mood swings with the low moods more common than the better moods

- Your muscles begin to decrease

- Your bone density decreases (Osteoporosis is helped along by a decrease in IGF-1 levels)

- You are at a higher risk of heart disease, high blood pressure problems, and you can more easily take on a diabetic state

Your doctor can test you for growth hormone deficiencies including IGF-1 with a blood test. If your doctor doesn't see the need to do this but wants to treat your high blood pressure, diabetes symptoms, and depression with medicine before checking your HGH and IGF-1, get a second opinion from someone who understands the importance of balanced hormones.

Putting Your IGF-1 in Balance

A synthetic form of IGF-1 is available to help children who have FTT, *Failure to Thrive*, a growth condition where their bodies do not grow and mature normally.

For most of us, diet is the key. A high fat, high protein, smart carbs, no sugar lifestyle will go a long way towards restoring IGF-1 and related hormones.

Although you cannot stop the aging process, you certainly can speed it up through a bad diet. Focus on organic produce, grass-fed beef, cage-free poultry and eggs, and raw, whole milk to slow down the act of aging. Moderate exercise also seems to work to help stave off brain-related disorders and aspects of aging. As a matter of fact, Dr. Eric Braverman, from Weill Cornell Medical College, has shown that increasing IGF-1 actually can reverse some of the serious problems that a lack of IGF-1 causes and can add protection against Alzheimer's disease.

SUMMARY

So there you have it. Fix your hormones if you want a healthy body and you want to be at your best weight.

"Hormones first" works best. You'll rarely do your body much good if you work on your weight first. You will be working against yourself, going against the grain (did you catch that pun?) or pushing a boulder uphill to use analogous phrases. Your hormones simply won't let you lose weight and keep it off until you balance them.

Fix your hormone levels first and let them *help you* fix your body and weight.

Can we be specific once more before the book ends? Here are some of the potential benefits that occur when your hormones go back into balance after being messed up:

- Your metabolism speeds up

- You lose weight without going hungry

- You eat more foods and still lose weight

- You are less likely to get diabetes

- You are less likely to get pre-diabetes

- You are less likely to get heart disease

- You are less likely to get cancer

- You will be happier

- You will look younger

- You will improve your vision

- You will have better skin and hair

- You are less likely to get wrinkles

- Your bones and nails will be strengthened

- You'll have a sex drive

- You'll have more energy

- You will delay the aging process

- You will live longer.

So what are you waiting for? Ditch all your processed food, buy only organic produce, grass fed beef, cage-free chicken and eggs, raw, whole milk, and lots of good oils and nuts and seeds.

Over or Under

If you're overweight, balancing your hormones will help because your hormones will work to get the excess weight off as quickly as possible. If you're underweight, balancing your hormones will help because your hormones will work to put on needed weight as quickly as possible.

We presented you with a lot of options in this book. The core thing to remember is that if you are having problems losing weight and feeling energetic even though you "eat well" and exercise a lot, then maybe diet and exercise aren't the most important problems holding you back from losing weight and feeling great.

If you feel bad or are overweight... the problem is most likely a hormonal imbalance.

Diet, Exercise, and Lifestyle Always Trump Drugs If Possible

Fortunately, your hormones are often fixed easily through diet and exercise. And even though you've been *trying* to lose weight through diet and exercise all this time, it needs to be a hormone-healthy diet and exercise to repair the hormone production and impair your weight gain.

Our advice is simple.

Incorporate the diet and exercise advice in this book, but concentrate on your hormones for the next month or two. Find a nutritionist in your area who can order blood tests, especially if you're feeling fatigued, have sexual issues, or can't seem to lose weight for the long-term. The nutritionist can help narrow down the hormones you may need to work on more closely.

With a balanced and healthy hormonal system, the exercise and diet will have an easier time helping you to lose weight.

Better quality food sources suggested in this book tend to cost more money than fast food joints and traditional grocery store packaged food. There is no getting around that.

Always stack your advantages. If you're going to add fats to your body (and you should), do it through organic nuts and seeds and healthy oils such as macadamia nut oil, extra virgin olive oil, extra virgin coconut oil, cod liver oil, as well as real butter. If you're going to add protein to your diet (and you should), do it through grass-fed beef, raw, whole milk from cows that were never given growth hormones, poultry and eggs from free-range chickens (even Walmart sells cage-free organic eggs from time to time!). Eat plenty of fibrous and colorful vegetables. Limit your intake of fruit to once a day or so at the most and try to stick with organic berries until your weight gets far more in balance due to balanced hormones.

Your Hormones and Health

I'm sure your health, as well as how you look and how you feel, is important to you or you wouldn't be reading this book. For various reasons people around the world are becoming fatter and unhealthier with each passing year. The medical costs associated with that are expensive. Why not pay a little bit more now for truly healthy foods and supplements and in the meantime live a higher quality life rather than spending more later on medical bills while dragging on through life with too many pounds and too little energy?

If you want to lose weight as fast as possible while saving money in the process, consider using Jennifer's *1 Day Diet*. That diet will work great in combination with the diet and other information in this book and the cost savings from being on the *1 Day Diet* helps you offset the costs of the higher quality foods recommended in this book. Good luck!

Sincerely,

Jennifer Jolan and Rich Bryda

COPYRIGHT AND TRADEMARK NOTICES

LIMITS OF LIABILITY & DISCLAIMERS OF WARRANTIES

substitute for direct, personal, professional medical care and diagnosis. None of the exercises or treatments (including products and services) mentioned in this book should be performed or otherwise used without clearance from your physician or health care provider. There may be risks associated with participating in activities or using products mentioned in this book for people in poor health or with pre-existing physical or mental health conditions.

Because these risks exist, you will not use such products or participate in such activities if you are in poor health or have a pre-existing mental or physical condition. If you choose to participate in these risks, you do so of your own free will and accord, knowingly and voluntarily assuming all risks associated with such activities. The materials in this book are provided "as is" and without warranties of any kind either express or implied. The Author disclaims all warranties, express or implied, including, but not limited to, implied warranties of merchantability and fitness for a particular purpose. The Author does not warrant that defects will be corrected, or that that the site or the server that makes this book available are free of viruses or other harmful components. The Author does not warrant or make any representations regarding the use or the results of the use of the materials in this book in terms of their correctness, accuracy, reliability, or otherwise. Applicable law may not allow the exclusion of implied warranties, so the above exclusion may not apply to you.

Under no circumstances, including, but not limited to, negligence, shall the Author be liable for any special or consequential damages that result from the use of, or the inability to use this book, even if the Author or his authorized representative has been advised of the possibility of such damages. Applicable law may not allow the limitation or exclusion of liability or incidental or consequential damages, so the above limitation or exclusion may not apply to you. In no event shall the Author's total liability to you for all damages, losses, and causes of action (whether in contract, tort, including but not limited to, negligence or otherwise) exceed the amount paid by you, if any, for this book. You agree to hold the Author of this book, the Author's owners, agents, affiliates, and employees harmless from any and all liability for all claims for damages due to injuries, including attorney fees and costs, incurred by you or caused to third parties by you, arising out of the products, services, and activities discussed in this book, excepting only claims for gross negligence or intentional tort.

You agree that any and all claims for gross negligence or intentional tort shall be settled solely by confidential binding arbitration per the American Arbitration Association's commercial arbitration rules. All arbitration must occur in the municipality where the Author's principal place of business is located. Arbitration fees and costs shall be split equally, and you are solely responsible for your own lawyer fees. Facts and information are believed to be accurate at the time they were placed in this book. All data provided in this book is to be used for information purposes only. The information contained within is not intended to provide specific physical or mental health advice, or any other advice whatsoever, for any individual or company and should not be relied upon in that regard. The services described are only offered in jurisdictions where they may be legally offered. Information provided is not all-inclusive, and is limited to information that is made available and such information should not be relied upon as all-inclusive or accurate. For more information about this policy, please contact the Author at the e-mail address listed in the Copyright Notice for this book.

IF YOU DO NOT AGREE WITH THESE TERMS AND EXPRESS CONDITIONS, DO NOT READ THIS BOOK. YOUR USE OF THIS BOOK, PRODUCTS, SERVICES, AND ANY PARTICIPATION IN ACTIVITIES MENTIONED ON THIS BOOK, MEAN THAT YOU ARE AGREEING TO BE LEGALLY BOUND BY THESE TERMS.

5834577R00090

Printed in Great Britain
by Amazon.co.uk, Ltd.,
Marston Gate.